BRAGG

APPLE CIDER VINEGAR

MIRACLE HEALTH SYSTEM

with the

BRAGG HEALTHY LIFESTYLE

Blueprint for Physical, Mental and Spiritual Improvement – Healthy, Vital Living to 120

Genesis 6:3

PAUL C. BRAGG, N.D., Ph.D.
LIFE EXTENSION SPECIALIST

and

PATRICIA BRAGG, N.D., Ph.D.
HEALTH & FITNESS EXPERT

Health   Peace
Happiness   Youthfulness
Love   Joy
Praise   Patience
Vitality   Fortitude
Strength   Charity
Faith

BECOME

A Bragg Health Crusader – for a 100% Healthy World for All!

HEALTH SCIENCE

Box 7, Santa Barbara, California 93102 USA

World Wide Web: www.bragg.com

Notice: Our writings are to help guide you to live a healthy lifestyle and prevent health problems. If you suspect you have a health problem, please seek qualified health professionals to help you make the healthiest informed choices. Diabetics should fast only under a health professional's supervision! If hypoglycemic, add spirulina or barley green powder to liquids when fasting.

BRAGG
APPLE CIDER
VINEGAR

MIRACLE HEALTH SYSTEM

PAUL C. BRAGG, N.D., Ph.D.
LIFE EXTENSION SPECIALIST
and
PATRICIA BRAGG, N.D., Ph.D.
HEALTH & FITNESS EXPERT

Health Science, Box 7, Santa Barbara, California 93102
Telephone (805) 968-1020, FAX (805) 968-1001
e-mail address: books@bragg.com

Quantity Purchases: Companies, Professional Groups, Churches, Clubs, Fundraisers etc. Please contact our Special Sales Department.

**To see Bragg Books and products on-line,
visit our website: www.bragg.com**

♻ This book is printed on recycled, acid-free paper.
- REVISED AND EXPANDED -
Fifty-second Edition MMII
ISBN: 0-87790-044-2

Published in the United States
HEALTH SCIENCE, Box 7, Santa Barbara, California 93102 USA

PAUL C. BRAGG, N.D., Ph.D.
World's Leading Healthy Lifestyle Authority

Paul C. Bragg's daughter Patricia and their wonderful, healthy members of the Bragg *Longer Life, Health and Happiness Club* exercise daily on the beautiful Fort DeRussy lawn, at world famous Waikiki Beach in Honolulu, Hawaii. Membership is free and open to everyone who wishes to attend any morning – Monday through Saturday, from 9 to 10:30 am – for Bragg Super Power Breathing and Health and Fitness Exercises. On Saturday there are often health lectures on how to live a long, healthy life! The group averages 75 to 125 per day, depending on the season. From December to March it can go up to 150. Its dedicated leaders have been carrying on the class for over 30 years. Thousands have visited the club from around the world and carried the Bragg Health and Fitness Crusade to friends and relatives back home. When you visit Honolulu, Hawaii, Patricia invites you and your friends to join her and the club for wholesome, healthy fellowship. She also recommends you visit the outer Hawaiian Islands (Kauai, Hawaii, Maui, Molokai) for a fulfilling, healthy vacation.

To maintain good health, normal weight and increase the good life of radiant health, joy and happiness, the body must be exercised properly (stretching, walking, jogging, running, biking, swimming, deep breathing, good posture, etc.) and nourished wisely with healthy foods. – Paul C. Bragg

KEEP BIOLOGICALLY HEALTHY & YOUTHFUL WITH EXERCISE & GOOD NUTRITION

Always remember you have the following important reasons for following The Bragg Healthy Lifestyle:

- The ironclad laws of Mother Nature and God.
- Your common sense, which tells you that you are doing right.
- Your aim to make your health better and your life longer.
- Your resolve to prevent illness so that you may enjoy life.
- Make an art of healthy living; you will be youthful at any age.
- You will retain your faculties and be hale, hearty, active and useful far beyond the ordinary length of years.
- You will also possess superior mental and physical powers!

WANTED – For Robbing Health & Life

KILLER Saturated Fats   CHOKER Hydrogenated Fats
CLOGGER Salt   DEADEYED Devitalized Foods
DOPEY Caffeine   HARD WATER Inorganic Minerals
PLUGGER Frying Pan   JERKY Turbulent Emotions
DEATH-DEALER Drugs   CRAZY Alcohol
GREASY Obesity   SMOKY Tobacco
HOGGY Overeating   LOAFER Laziness

What Wise Men Say

Wisdom does not show itself so much in precept as in life – a firmness of mind and mastery of appetite. – Seneca

I saw few die of hunger – of eating, a hundred thousand. – Ben Franklin

Govern well thy appetite, lest Sin surprise thee, & her black attendant, Death. – Milton

The food shall be thy remedy. – Hippocrates

Our prayers should be for a sound mind in a healthy body. – Juvenal

Health is…a blessing that money cannot buy. – Izaak Walton

The natural healing force within us is the greatest force in getting well.
– Hippocrates, Father of Medicine

Of all the knowledge, that most worth having is the knowledge about health! The first requisite of a good life is to be a healthy person. – Herbert Spencer

Do You Show Signs of PREMATURE AGEING?

Is everything you do a big effort?

•

Have you started to lose your skin tone?
Muscle tone?

•

Do small things irritate you?
Are you forgetful?   Confused?

•

Have voices begun to fade?

•

Has your vision started to dim?

•

Do you wobble a little when you walk?

•

Do you get out of breath
when you climb stairs?

•

How limber is your back?

•

Do your joints creak?

•

How well do you adjust to cold and heat?

•

Ask yourself this important question:
Do I seem to be slipping and
not quite like myself anymore?
If the answer to this question is "Yes,"
You had better do something about it!

START TODAY
Living The
Bragg Healthy
Lifestyle!

He who understands Mother Nature walks with God. – Edgar Cayce

v

BRAGG HEALTH CRUSADES for 21st Century
Teaching People Worldwide to Live Healthy, Happy, Stronger, Longer Lives for a Better World

We love sharing, teaching and giving world-wide, and you can share this love by being a partner by sharing The Bragg Health Crusades message. We are dedicated with a passion to help others! We feel blessed when you and your family's lives improve through following our teachings from the Bragg Health Books and The Bragg Crusades. It makes our years of faithful service so worthwhile! We will keep sharing, and please do write us how our teachings have helped you.

The Miracle of Fasting book has been the #1 book for 15 years in Russia! Why? Because we show them how to live a healthy, wholesome life for less money, and it's so easy to understand and follow. Most healthful lifestyle habits are free (good posture, clean thoughts, plain natural food, exercise and deep breathing, all of which promotes energy and health into the body). We continue to reach the multitudes worldwide with our health books and teachings, lectures, crusades, radio and TV outreaches.

My joy and priorities come from God, Mother Nature and healthy living. I love being a health crusader and spreading health worldwide, for now it's needed more than ever! My father and I also pioneered Health TV with our program "Health and Happiness" from Hollywood. Yes – it's thrilling to be a Health Crusader and you will enjoy it also. See back pages to list names (yourself, family and friends) who you feel would benefit from receiving our free Health Bulletins!

By reading Bragg Self-Health Books you gain a new confidence that you can help yourself, family and friends to The Bragg Healthy Principles of Living! Please call your local book stores and health stores and ask for the Bragg Health Books. Prayerfully, we hope to have all stores stock the Bragg Books. We do keep prices as low as possible so they will be affordable and available for everyone to learn to live and enjoy a healthier, happier and longer life!

With Blessings of Health, Peace and Love,

Patricia Bragg

BRAGG HEALTH CRUSADES, America's Health Pioneers
Keep Bragg Health Crusades "Crusading" with your tax deductible donations.
7340 Hollister Ave., Santa Barbara, CA 93117 USA (805) 968-1020
Spreading health worldwide since 1912

Contents

In 400 B.C., Hippocrates, the Father of Medicine, treated his patients with amazing raw Apple Cider Vinegar because he recognized its powerful cleansing and healing qualities. It's a naturally occurring antibiotic and antiseptic that fights germs and bacteria.

Title

*"Open thou thine eyes, that I may behold
wondrous things out of thy law."* – Psalms 119:18

Astronomers Find Vinegar in Distant Space

In a stellar cloud 25,000 light years from Earth, researchers recently found organic vinegar, a molecule that may have played a big role in the formation of life. – University of Chicago. See www.admin.uiuc.edu/NB/96.06/10vinegar.html

Contents

*When you sell a man a book you don't just sell him paper, ink and glue,
you sell him a whole new life! There's heaven and earth in a real book.
The real purpose of books is to inspire the mind to do its own thinking!*
– Christopher Morely

Contents

Doubt destroys. Faith builds! – Robert Collier

*The natural healing force within us is the greatest
force in getting well.* – Hippocrates, Father of Medicine

*When health is absent, wisdom cannot reveal itself, art
cannot become manifest, strength cannot be exerted. Wealth
is useless, and reason is powerless.* – Herophiles, 300 B.C.

TEN HEALTH COMMANDMENTS

Thou shall respect and protect thy body as the highest manifestation of life.

Thou shall abstain from all unnatural, devitalized food and stimulating beverages.

Thou shall nourish thy body with only Natural unprocessed, live foods, that . . .

Thou shall extend thy years in health for loving, sharing with others and charitable service.

Thou shall regenerate thy body by the right balance of activity and rest.

Thou shall purify thy cells, tissues and blood with healthy foods, pure water, fresh air and sunshine.

Thou shall abstain from all food when out of sorts in mind or body.

Thou shall keep all thoughts, words and emotions pure, good, calm, kind, uplifting and loving.

Thou shall increase thy knowledge of Nature's Laws, follow them and enjoy the fruits of thy life's labor.

Thou shall lift up thyself, friends and family by obedience to God's Healthy, Pure Laws of Living.

Paul C. Bragg and *Patricia Bragg*

*Teach me Thy way O Lord, and
lead me in a simple plain path. – Psalms 27:11*

---

*And Jesus full of the Holy Ghost returned from Jordan and was lead
by the Spirit into the wilderness. Jesus fasted for 40 days and after
the fast He gave His famous Sermon on the Mount. – Luke 4:1-2*

✿❀ Bragg Healthy Lifestyle Plan ❀✿

- *Read, plan, plot, and follow through for supreme health and longevity.*
- *Underline, highlight or dog-ear pages as you read important passages.*
- *Organizing your lifestyle helps you identify what's important in your life.*
- *Be faithful to your health goals everyday for a healthy, long, happy life.*
- *Where space allows we have included "words of wisdom" from great minds to motivate and inspire you. Please share your favorite sayings with us.*
- *Do write us about your successes following The Bragg Vinegar Program.*

Bragg
Apple Cider Vinegar
Miracle Health System

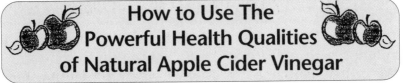

How to Use The Powerful Health Qualities of Natural Apple Cider Vinegar

Research worldwide supports and commends what Hippocrates (the father of medicine) found and treated his patients with in 400 B.C. He discovered that natural, undistilled Apple Cider Vinegar (or ACV)* is a powerful cleansing and healing elixir – a naturally occurring antibiotic and antiseptic that fights germs and bacteria – for a healthier, stronger, longer life!

The versatility of ACV as a powerful body cleansing agent is legendary. It's been traced to Egyptian urns as far back as 3000 B.C. The Babylonians used it as a condiment and preservative, while Julius Caesar's army used ACV tonic to stay healthy and fight off disease. The Greeks and Romans kept vinegar vessels for healing and flavoring. It was used in Biblical times as an antiseptic and a healing agent and is mentioned in the Bible. In Paris in the Middle Ages it was sold from barrels by street vendors as a body deodorant, healing tonic and delicious vinegar drink to keep the body healthy and ageless.

Even Christopher Columbus and crew on his voyage to discover America in 1492 had vinegar barrels for prevention of scurvy as did U.S. Civil war soldiers. It helped disinfect and heal their wounds. For centuries in Japan, the feared Samurai warriors drank it for strength and power. ACV has been used for thousands of years not only for health reasons, but as a cleansing agent to remove bacteria, germs, odors, and even stains and spots.

1

A teacher for the day can be a guiding light for a lifetime!
Bragg books are silent health teachers – never tiring, ready night or day to help you help yourself to health! Our books are written with love and a deep desire to guide you to a healthy lifestyle. – Patricia Bragg

*The best is the organic, raw, unfiltered, unpasteurized apple cider vinegar with the "mother," available most Health Stores. See back pages for info.

Natural (undistilled) organic, raw ACV can really be called one of Mother Nature's most perfect foods. It is made from fresh, crushed apples which are then allowed to mature naturally in wooden barrels, as wood seems to "boost" the natural fermentation. Natural ACV should be a rich, brownish color and if held to the light you might see a tiny formation of "cobweb-like" substances we call the miracle "mother". Usually some "mother" shows at bottom of bottle as it ages more. It never needs refrigeration. You can also save some "mother" and transfer it to work in other natural vinegars. When you smell natural ACV, there's a pungent odor and sometimes it's so ripened it puckers your mouth and smarts your eyes – these are natural, good signs.

Why Has Natural Apple Cider Vinegar Disappeared from Grocers' Shelves?

The blame for the disappearance of natural raw apple cider vinegar from supermarkets lies on the shoulders of the general public, as well as the producers of vinegar.

Most people buy food with their eyes, not thinking of good nutrition. Vinegar producers failed to enlighten the public on what powerful health qualities are locked within natural ACV. Why? Because they didn't have the slightest knowledge of the health values of natural, raw, organic, unfiltered, cloudy (to some, less attractive-looking) ACV with the "mother". They produced pasteurized, refined, distilled vinegars because the public demanded it. It was simply filling current supply and demand that tragically removed the priceless miraculous health benefits.

Powerful Health Qualities Removed

You cannot completely blame the producers of vinegar. They are not nutritionists, nor are they biochemists. Their business is to give the customers what they want. Most people purchase vinegar for flavoring, also for pickling and marinating their foods. Some women use it to rinse their hair after shampooing, as it leaves it squeaky clean, softer and much easier to manage.

ACV is also a great germ fighter in the home, lab, etc.. Some mix it with water to wash windows, as it removes sludge and keeps them sparkling clean, as it does for the body. ACV has hundreds of uses and its versatility is legendary as a powerful household cleansing and deodorizing agent free of dangerous chemicals. (See vinegar cleaning hints – pages 103 to 105.)

ACV Has Proven Powerful Health Qualities

Both the general public and the producers of vinegar have been uninformed as to the powerful health qualities of organic, raw, unfiltered, fully ripened ACV. Ignorance isn't always bliss! When most people see natural apple cider vinegar with the brownish color and the tiny, cobweb "mother" floating in it, they think it looks unappetizing. The general public has been educated and brainwashed to want everything they purchase to have perfect eye appeal!

To meet this demand that vinegar must be clear and light colored and free from the brownish, cobweb "mother" is the reason producers distill their vinegar. In distilling, the vinegar is turned to steam by heating. Therefore it destroys the powerful enzymes and distills out the life-giving minerals such as potassium, phosphorus, natural organic sodium, magnesium, sulphur, iron, copper, natural organic fluorine, silicon, trace minerals, essential amino acids and pectin and many other powerful nutrients! Distilling also destroys the natural malic and tartaric acids which are important in fighting body toxins and inhibiting unfriendly bacteria.

You can see how the public, with their obsession for *eye appeal foods,* reacts. The producers of apple cider vinegar, who agreed to sell their product for a profit, put a "death warrant" against healthy, organic, raw, fully ripened ACV. The public got what they wanted – a clear, appealing, but dead ACV. When natural ACV was hard to find, other strange vinegars began to appear on grocery shelves. The first was malt vinegar, a refined vinegar. It's clear and acceptable to the public. It tastes like vinegar, but has none of the healing qualities of natural, raw ACV.

The universally accepted #1 fruit, the apple, is popular across America and around the world. Early American settlers, the Pilgrims, brought apples to America in the 1600s and became Johnny Appleseeders, starting apple orchards that eventually spread throughout America.

Commercial Vinegars are Real Tragedies

Then came the real tragedy: a food chemist produced an imitation vinegar from coal tar! It looked clean, white and tasted like vinegar. Today it's the most popular vinegar in supermarkets. It's cheaper than distilled vinegar or malt vinegar. Most people buy these worthless vinegars. There's nothing good about commercial vinegars, except they look clean and taste like vinegar. They have no health value! They don't contain the health values of organic, raw ACV with the *mother*. Sad fact: millions worldwide never get the health benefits of this natural organic apple cider vinegar as Hippocrates used in 400 B.C.

Millions Suffer from Malnutrition

"Mal" means bad. As a consequence of not getting natural, healthy, balanced diets, millions worldwide suffer from many forms of subclinical malnutrition. This means many people, due to vitamin and mineral deficiencies, feel half-sick most of the time! They lack vim, vigor and "Go Power" and feel tired most of the time. Their daily food intake and the commercial vinegars they use don't provide sufficient vitamins and minerals, nor the potassium their bodies require. They lack vital power and feel exhausted. This is the reason people turn to stimulants like coffee, America's most popular unhealthy drink, and to colas, alcohol, cigarettes and over-the-counter "fix-all" drugs. After these stimulants' effects wear off, they feel terrible. They just exist, and are not living happy, healthy lives!

Coffee – America's #1 Drug Addiction

Coffee drinking (caffeine) is the #1 drug addiction in America! Millions of pounds of coffee are sold to America yearly. That's not to mention the caffeine in soft drinks. Plus there's millions of addicted chocoholics who are hooked on chocolate and sugar – a harmful combination. The shocking list of caffeine-related side effects include: high blood pressure, hypertension, arrythmia, elevated cholesterol, glucose, increased tendencies to allergies, chronic fatigue and autoimmune disorders, etc.

Man is fully responsible for his nature and his choices. – Jean-Paul Sartre

You see these unhappy people about you every day. They are washed out and ageing prematurely. Many lack skin and muscle tone and have dark circles and puffy (water) bags under their eyes. Their eyes lose the sparkle of health and youthfulness and become like dead fish eyes. Malnourished people are mostly lifeless and everything they do requires a tremendous effort. They are not really living and most are not happy. Many suffer from depression and mental fatigue – nerve burnout.

Apples Are Rich in Potassium & Enzymes

"An apple a day keeps the doctor away" is a familiar saying to millions. It carries good common sense. The apple is one of God's great health-giving foods.

Apples are a rich source of potassium, which is to the soft tissues of the body as calcium is to the bones and harder tissues. Potassium is the mineral of youthfulness; it is the "artery softener," keeping the arteries of the body flexible and resilient. It is a fighter of dangerous bacteria and viruses. Yes, when you say, "An apple a day keeps the doctor away," you are talking good, down-to-earth old-fashioned folk medicine for vibrant, life-long health!

The apple has stood the test of time. It is one of the oldest known fruits that humans consume. Since the Garden of Eden the apple has played a vital part in our destiny. People have been eating apples for thousands of years. Apple eaters have a certain healthfulness that non-apple eaters never achieve.

Apples are delicious fruits that most people enjoy eating, but we look on the apple as more than something good to eat. Potassium is the key mineral in the constellation of minerals; it's so important to every living thing that without it there would be no life!

Most humans are deficient in potassium (page 15) and it reflects in their cell tissues and throughout their entire body. Look around you. How many people do you see that have the super glow of health?

There is no wealth greater than the health of the body. – The Bible

Millions Suffer From Potassium Deficiency

Millions living in today's civilization and eating its commercialized, processed foods have a potassium deficiency. The skin and muscle tone are bad. The flesh does not cling firmly to the body's bony framework. Lines and wrinkles fill the face and neck.

One sign is flabby, excess skin hanging over the eyes. If the potassium deficiency continues, the prolapsing eyelids progress. Soon, people are looking out of little slits instead of wide-open eyes. Thousands have turned to eyelid surgery to correct droopy eyelids, also called hooded eyelids, that roll down and rest on their eyelashes causing eyestrain, headaches, etc. If an eye doctor suggests corrective surgery for this, the insurance company usually honors the claim. It's an in/out local procedure. It's best the eye surgeon is board certified. People wrongly blame their age for their droopy eyelids, skin changes and lack of muscle tone.

But the truth is . . . you must have potassium to build and maintain youthful, healthy tissues! If you don't get required amount of potassium daily, you soon acquire an old-age look and feel. This premature ageing is usually due to potassium deficiency and unhealthy living!

It is the same in your flower and vegetable garden. Potassium is necessary for the production of the substances that give rigidity to plant stems and increase their resistance to the many diseases that attack plants. Potassium is also the powerful element that changes seeds into plants and beautiful flowers by progressive development. If plants become deficient in potassium, they stop their growth. If the potassium deficiency is not corrected, the plant slowly starts to wither, turns yellow and dies! The same is true of animals and humans with a potassium deficiency: there is a slow degeneration leading to death of the cells, then death of life.

Every day the average heart, your best friend, beats 100,000 times and pumps 2,000 gallons of blood for nourishing your body. In about 70 years that adds up to more than 360 million (faithful) heartbeats. Please be good to your heart and live The Bragg Healthy Lifestyle for a long, happy, healthy life! Here's to Genesis 6:3 for you. – Patricia Bragg

Refined Foods & Flours Remove Vital Potassium which Causes Poor Health!

Robbed grains: The miller refines and processes our grains to get white flour that will keep for years . . . that becomes the staff of death! Even bugs have more sense – they won't eat it because it has been robbed of its potassium and vital life-giving qualities!

Shocking loss of potassium and nutrients in making white flour: In milling wheat, the miller refines out 25 important food elements, including vital amino acids, vitamin E, bran, the rich B-complex vitamins and potassium. Cows fed refined grain, with the potassium milled out and de-germed, die early of heart failure.

The more they refine vital potassium out of foods, the sicker Americans get: People waste money, time, and energy and suffer the loss of health by being sick. The #1 health plan should be to teach Americans how to live a healthy lifestyle that maintains health by correct eating and living habits. Healthy nutrition will create bones that last a lifetime, cells that resist disease and arteries that stay healthy, cholesterol-free and unclogged!

Bad Nutrition –
#1 Cause of Sickness
"Diet-related diseases account for 68% of all deaths."
– Dr. C. Everett Koop

Dr. Koop & Patricia

America's former Surgeon General and our friend, said this in his famous 1988 landmark report on nutrition and health in America. People don't die of infectious conditions as such, but of malnutrition that allows the germs to get a foothold in sickly bodies. Also, bad nutrition is usually the main cause of noninfectious, fatal or degenerative conditions. When the body has its full vitamin and mineral quota, including precious potassium, it's almost impossible for germs to get a foothold in a healthy, powerful bloodstream and tissues!

The Body Has the Seed of Eternal Life

Outside of fatal accidents, there is no reason why a person should leave before his or her time. It has been proven by some of the greatest scientific minds that there are no special diseases of old age. A person should not die simply because they live to 60, 70, 80 or 90 years of age, because calendar age is not toxic. People create their toxins by their eating and living habits.

Most people die of some fatal condition that they have built into their bodies by incorrect living or by violating the natural laws that govern the physical body.

The two great enemies of life are toxic poisons (found in some foods, air, water and soil) and the nutritional deficiencies caused by unhealthy diet. The best prevention of sickness is to eat vital, healthy foods (organic is best and safer), especially those high in potassium. These provide the body with correct, life-giving nourishment.

Every 90 days a new bloodstream, the river of life, is built in the body by the foods you eat, the liquids you drink and the air you breathe. From the bloodstream the body's cells are made, nourished and maintained. Every 11 months we have a new set of billions of miraculous body cells, and every 2 years we have an entirely new set of bones and hard tissues. There is no reason to get old because the body is constantly cleansing and renewing its cells to keep your precious human temple healthy for life.

Nutrition directly affects growth, development, reproduction and well-being of an individual's physical and mental condition. Health depends upon nutrition more than on any other single factor. – Dr. Wm. H. Sebrell, Jr.

Laws of health are inexorable; we see people going down and out in their prime of life because no attention is paid to them! – Paul Bragg

---

Age does not depend upon years, but upon temperament and health.

Your Daily Habits Form Your Future

Habits can be wrong, good or bad, healthy or unhealthy, rewarding or unrewarding. The right or wrong habits, decisions, actions, words or deeds . . . are up to you! Wisely choose your habits, as they can make or break your life! – Patricia Bragg

Exercise Helps Keep You More Youthful, Healthier, Stronger, Flexible and Trim

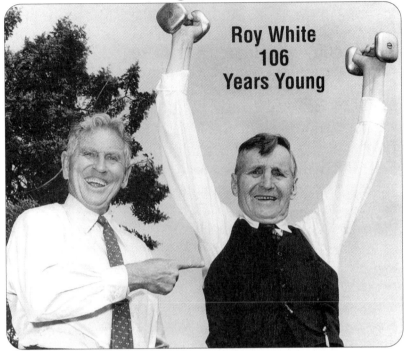

Roy White
106
Years Young

9

Paul C. Bragg and His Health Follower, Roy White

Paul and Roy practiced progressive weight training 3 times a week to stay healthy and fit. Scientists have proven that weight training works miracles for all ages by maintaining more flexibility, energy and youthful stamina!

See pages 88-90 for some of the amazing scientific data coming in from around the world on the important longevity, health, renewing and rewarding benefits of regular exercise and living a healthy lifestyle!

Never shatter someone else's dreams or hopes;
these are as precious, and as rare, as life itself.

Man is the sole and absolute master of his own fate forever.
What he has sown in the times of his ignorance, he must
inevitably reap; when he attains enlightenment, it is for him to
sow what he chooses and reap accordingly. – Geraldine Coster

Change your mind and change your life.

Dream big, think big, but enjoy the small miracles of everyday life!

Dr. Carrel's Eternal Life Successful Study

Nobel Scientist Dr. Alexis Carrel of the Rockefeller Institute in New York in 1912 kept the cells of an embryo chicken heart alive and healthy for over 35 years by daily monitoring its complete nutrition, cleansing and elimination. A chicken's lifespan averages 7 years!

Apple cider vinegar was given to the chicken embryo daily for its full quota of potassium. Dr. Carrel definitively proved to the entire world that the body has a seed of eternal life. He could have continued this experiment indefinitely to give the embryo immortality, but felt 35 years proved the point that man kills himself by his wrong habits of overeating and living an unhealthy lifestyle. This study showed us the importance of nutrition, cleansing and apple cider vinegar to life, health and longevity!

Web: *nobel.sdsc.edu/medicine/laureates/1912/carrel-bio.html*

Recently a remarkable study on longevity was done with earthworms. By monitoring their food intake, then decreasing it to only what was nutritionally necessary, these worms multiplied their lifespan (see bottom page 55). The results from these and many other studies have revealed the key to longer life. Many scientists know no reason why these same principles could not apply to everyone. Even today the Hunzas of Kashmir and the Georgians of Russia lead active lives to 120 and older!

Potassium Deficiency Can Stunt Growth

We have enjoyed making over 10 scientific health expeditions throughout the world, studying the health, longevity and growth of various races of people. We found areas where the topsoil was deficient in potassium and the people living off foods grown from this potassium-deficient soil were prone to be stunted in growth and have a shorter lifespan. The pygmies of Africa are stunted and short-lived. The same is true of the Arctic Eskimos. In their daily diet, they just do not get the required amount of potassium and other minerals that are so important to growth, health and long life.

The strongest principle of growth lies in the human choice. – George Elliot

Mentally Handicapped Children and Adults Suffer from Potassium Deficiency

We have closely studied the relationship between mentally handicapped children and adults and potassium deficiency. Many years ago, my dad brought three of these children to our home for study and observation. Three times daily – in morning, noon and night – the children had the ACV drink (1 tsp. ACV and 1 tsp. raw honey in glass of distilled water, both rich in potassium). Dad put the children on The Bragg Healthy Lifestyle which gave them extra amounts of wonderful potassium. Daily they were given multiple vitamin-mineral supplements and some niacin (50 mgs – vitamin B-3). In 3 weeks, these children became more mentally alert. After living in our home for less than a year, they were able to resume their schooling with children their own age!

Another amazing study – we brought three mentally handicapped adults into our home and after putting them on the ACV routine plus living The Bragg Healthy Lifestyle, they became self-supporting in less than a year!

Potassium Deficiency Produces Senility

Throughout the world, there are millions of senile, prematurely old people. Many don't know their own names, nor can they recognize their family or closest friends. They are just barely existing. It might seem that they have degenerated so much that it's almost a hopeless task to try to save them, but please try! We feel they can be restored to useful lives if the toxic poisons are flushed from their bodies and their nutritional deficiencies (nutrients, potassium pg 15, and niacin, etc.) are corrected!

Be a Shining Star . . . *Rise above any problems – you are not locked into unhealthy habits – remember you are the captain and can guide your being into a fresh, exciting, new life filled with wonderful challenges, so get ready to take off for Super Health on Earth!* – Patricia Bragg

We choose our joys and sorrows before we experience them. – Kahlil Gibran

You can change and improve the quality of your health by detoxifying your body. Start Your Bragg Healthy Lifestyle today!

Miracles with Potassium

Years ago, we selected four senile people we felt could be helped. We put them on The Bragg Healthy Lifestyle with the ACV drink and healthy foods rich in potassium. Out of the four, we were able to save three of them. All three left the convalescent home where they had been confined and became healthy, happy and self-sufficient. Two of them made remarkable recoveries. One went back to contracting and building at 83, and the other in his mid 80s resumed his accounting career!

Most senile people suffer from a clogged arterial system. Potassium is to the soft tissues of the body as calcium is to the hard structures. The potassium goes into the clogged, caked arteries and cleans out the rust and dirt just like vinegar water removes grime from windows. One can't think clearly if the arteries are heavily clogged with cholesterol and toxic poisons.

Potassium might be called the great detergent of the arteries. Potassium slows down the hardening and clogging processes that cause deadly harm to the whole cardiovascular system. Organic, raw ACV contains the miraculous potassium that makes the flesh of farm animals healthier and more tender. There is very little doubt, in animal and man, that the main function of potassium is to keep the tissues healthy, soft and pliable, and to help prevent heart attacks and strokes!

Paul Bragg Talks about Vinegar Miracles on His Family's Farm in His Youth

Long years of research have proven to me that natural apple cider vinegar is a potent source of potassium. I was raised on a large farm. On this farm, we grew many varieties of apples. I was a great apple eater. Each year my father made natural apple cider vinegar and stored it in wooden barrels. On our table we used this natural apple cider vinegar and our large family loved it.

Potassium is the key mineral in the constellation of minerals; it's so important to every living thing that without it there would be no life. Bragg's Organic Apple Cider Vinegar is a rich source of potassium.

ACV Relieves Chronic Fatigue

My father was a splendid farmer and many times I would watch him add ACV to the feed and water of ailing animals (cattle, horses, sheep, dogs, cats, etc.) and it acted like magic. ACV seemed to possess some miracle ingredient that helped restore health to the animals.*

The nearest doctor was 32 miles from our home. If a doctor was needed, he had to come by horse and buggy over miles of rough, dirt roads. So, at our home we developed simple self-health remedies and apple cider vinegar played an important health role.

I remember when my father would put in long hours at the farm during the harvest period. He was up long before daybreak and didn't retire until late at night. I would watch him come into the kitchen, put 2 heaping tsps. of honey in a glass, add 2 tsps. of raw apple cider vinegar, fill the glass with water and then sip it slowly.

I would ask, "Father, why do you drink apple cider vinegar, honey and water?" Father would reply, "Son, farm work is long, hard work. It can produce extreme body fatigue. Whatever is in this apple cider vinegar and honey drink relieves me of that chronic fatigue."

Father was definitely correct. There was an ingredient in that drink that renewed his vitality and relieved him of the chronic fatigue and stiffness. That ingredient was potassium, along with the powerful enzymes, minerals and trace elements that are in organic, raw apple cider vinegar.

Most people today, when they work hard, turn to all kinds of dangerous stimulants to relieve their chronic fatigue: alcohol, tea, coffee, cola drinks and pep pills and other dangerous, addictive drugs.

My father's good advice fell on youthful ears. It was some years later that I realized that my father was a smart man in using raw honey and raw apple cider vinegar, rich in potassium, to combat chronic fatigue.

---

*ACV helps animals stay healthy. Mixture: *1 cup ACV with 3 cups distilled water. Once daily in feed or water: for small animals, add 1 tsp. ACV mixture; for large animals, add 2 to 3 tsps. Or administer orally with eye dropper, baster or squeeze bottle. To relieve skin rashes or itching apply topically. Add to bath or rinse water to keep skin healthy and ward off fleas. (We have had testimonials of praise in various horse and dog magazines.)*

Unhealthy Diet Brings Sickness

At 12, I was sent from my rugged farm life to an expensive military academy as a gift for saving a wealthy man from drowning. That institution's food gradually broke my health! The unhealthy diet of sugared, refined, overcooked and dead foods served there ruined my health. It made me the victim of a consuming disease, tuberculosis.

At no time did I see our wonderful ACV or raw honey at the table of the military academy. It was not until I met the great healer Dr. Rollier at his health sanitarium in Switzerland, where I regained my health, that I again came in contact with the miracles of ACV and *honey, both rich in essential potassium! I owe much of my recovery to apple cider vinegar and honey, as they are persistent fighters against germs and toxins! Each morning, I was given the same drink my father took for energy and health. Dr. Rollier urged us to put apple cider vinegar on all of our raw vegetable salads and steamed greens. He also urged us to eat an abundance of raw vegetables and fresh fruits each day as they are Mother Nature's purifiers. He was a wise doctor and knew how valuable potassium and raw fruits and vegetables are for maintaining 100% health.

I was 100% cured from TB in less than 2 years after cleansing and rebuilding myself with a balanced natural diet, correct deep breathing, exercise and Alpine sunshine. Healthy living was my cure! I have been an ardent user of organic, raw ACV and raw honey ever since. In our Bragg health teachings and writings we have always advocated the use of this miraculous source of potassium.

It was in Switzerland that I started to fulfill my earlier pledge to God, that if I recovered my health, I would become a health crusader and devote my life to sharing the message of health and wellness with the world! When I finished my schooling, I went on to full-time crusading for a healthier world! (See the Bragg Bio back pages.)

Raw honey has many miraculous nutrients (vitamins, potassium, enzymes, etc.). It's a natural occurring antibiotic and antiseptic. Ancient Egyptian medical documents touted honey as an essential natural cure-all, listing 500 honey remedies. Hippocrates, the father of medicine, prescribed honey because it fights bacteria, blocks infection, combats inflamation, reduces pain, improves circulation, stimulates regrowth of tissue, makes healing faster and reduces scarring. Apple Cider Vinegar and honey together are nature's perfect cure!

Body Signs of Potassium Deficiency

🍎 Bone and muscle aches and pains, especially lower back.

🍎 Shooting pains when straightening up after leaning over.

🍎 Dizziness upon straightening up after leaning over.

🍎 Morning dull headaches upon arising and when stressed.

🍎 The body feels heavy, tired and it's an effort to move.

🍎 Dull, faded-looking hair that lacks sheen and luster.

🍎 The scalp is itchy. Dandruff, premature hair thinning or some balding may occur.

🍎 The hair is unmanageable, mats, often looks straw-like, is sometimes extremely dry and other times oily.

🍎 The eyes itch, feel sore and uncomfortable, and appear bloodshot and watery. Also, eyelids may be granulated with white matter collecting in the corners.

🍎 The eyes tire easily and will not focus as they should.

🍎 Loss of mental alertness and onset of confusion, making decisions difficult. The memory fails, making you forget names and places you should easily remember.

🍎 You tire physically and mentally with the slightest effort.

🍎 You become easily irritable and impatient with your family, friends and loved ones, and even with your business and social acquaintances.

🍎 You feel nervous, depressed and in a mental fog. You have difficulty getting things done, due to mental and muscle and body fatigue. The slightest effort can leave you upset, nervous and trembling.

🍎 At times, your hands and feet get chilled, even in warm weather, which is a sign of potassium deficiency.

Potassium deficiency is a proven contributing cause of many illnesses, including:
Arthritis, kidney stones, atrial fibrillation, adrenal insufficiency, celiac disease, high blood pressure, coronary artery disease, ulcerative colitis, hypothyroidism, irritable bowel syndrome, Alzheimer's disease, multiple sclerosis, myasthenia gravis, Crohn's disease, lupus, atherosclerosis, diabetes and stroke. – Linda Page, N.D., Ph.D. *Healthy Healing*

Life is Thrilling When You Can Help Others!

I founded the health movement and originated, named and started the first Health Food Store. Then, through The Bragg Health Crusades, I inspired hundreds of Bragg students to open the first Health Food Stores in their areas across America and then worldwide. It's thrilling and rewarding to live a life of service helping and inspiring others to live a healthy lifestyle! God has blessed me!

Apple Cider Vinegar Miracle for Overweight

More than a third of Americans are trying to lose weight. Forty billion dollars are spent yearly on diet programs and products. Rather than a yo-yo diet, these people need The Bragg Healthy Lifestyle and ACV! Please understand ACV will not reduce a person who does not control their intake of food. But the ACV drink and a healthy diet of 1,200 calories daily, plus regular exercise will do miracles in reducing excess weight. Take the ACV drink 3 times daily. It consists of 1 to 2 tsps. equally of organic raw ACV and raw honey (optional) mixed in a glass of distilled water. Also the Diet Research Center in England reported, *"better reducing and firming with ACV daily massages* (mix 3 parts Bragg Organic ACV to 1 part Bragg Organic Olive Oil); helps the body reduce excess fat."*

16

Along with this healthy ACV drink, there must be a healthy reducing diet. (Read the Bragg *Miracle of Fasting* book for more reducing info.) This means that all refined, processed, sugared products and beverages and all dairy products are eliminated from your diet. The diet should consist of a wide variety of fresh organic fruits; raw salads; raw nuts and seeds; raw, steamed, baked or stir-fried vegetables; brown rice; tofu; beans; and whole grain pastas. Read our Bragg Recipe book for hundreds of delicious, healthy recipes, available most health & book stores, call & request them. If unavailable call (800)446-1990.

---

*Massages are soothing, relaxing and bring many beneficial healthy changes. They improve circulation and unclog body forces which helps promote healing and smoother, fit muscles. See pages 91 to 94.

Thermogenic herbs suppress appetite – barley grass, spirulina, alfalfa, sea vegetables, green drinks, etc. – taken with 500 mg of Carnitine and 200-400 mcg Chromium Picolinate promote weight loss and firming. Portion control meals, exercise and these herbs all help weight reduction.

Combatting Underweight

Apple cider vinegar is proving to be one of the greatest aids to health known to science. It's a 100% natural substance produced by powerful natural enzymes from healthy organic apples, free of any toxic chemicals.

The underweight person is usually deficient in these powerful enzymes and therefore cannot use or burn up the food that is put into their body. No matter how much fatty food, protein or any other kind of food is ingested, often it is not used properly by the body if important enzymes are missing. Enzyme deficiencies always cause problems! If underweight, drink the following ACV cocktail each morning upon arising: 2 tsps. ACV and 2 tsps. honey in a glass of distilled water. Add to this 2 drops of liquid iodine made from seaweed, available in Health Stores. This adds natural iodine, important to body health and helps normalize body weight up or down as needed. Then, with each meal take a multi-digestive enzyme (page 87) and always be faithful to The Bragg Healthy Lifestyle. Remember, healthy foods are needed body fuel to enjoy a long fulfilled life.

Purify Your Cells by Ridding
The Body of Dangerous Toxic Wastes

Toxic poisons are the cause of most troubles in the human body. Most people do not have sufficient vital force to supply the eliminative organs with the strength to remove normal waste from the body. The toxins remain and lodge in the joints and organs of the body. We have a name for each symptom that gives us pain and trouble. Certain toxic wastes that are harmful to the whole body are rendered harmless by a miraculous substance in organic, raw ACV with the powerful *mother*. Scientists call this protective action *acetolysis*.

In 400 B.C., Hippocrates, the Father of Medicine, treated his patients with amazing raw Apple Cider Vinegar because he recognized its powerful cleansing and healing qualities. It is a naturally occurring antibiotic and antiseptic that fights germs and bacteria.

A recent study showed people with large waistlines had shorter lifespans.

Caution: The Army Diet – what you overeat goes to the front.

Apple Cider Vinegar for Body Purification

It's time for life changes when you feel badly and don't seem to have the Human Go Power and Vital Force to do the things in life that are necessary! It's time to flush out the energy depleting, problem causing toxic wastes that are clogging your machinery and organs of elimination! Waste products broken down by this ACV process are flushed out. Remember, your important organs of elimination are the bowel, the lungs, the skin and the kidneys. They are your faithful servants! They work hard 24 hours a day to detox and flush out toxic wastes. Many times these eliminative organs need help and that is when the ACV drink comes to their aid!

Follow the ACV daily program. In addition, add 1 tsp. ACV to 6 ounces of salt-free tomato or fresh vegetable juice (carrot and greens) and drink between meals, daily. Be sure to do a cleansing fast (page 58) 1 day weekly and faithfully follow The Bragg Healthy Lifestyle, which is explained throughout the book in full, simple details.

Apple Cider Vinegar Relieves Headaches

People blame their headaches on many different organs of the body. Most headaches are blamed on the eyes, the nerves, the liver, the sinuses, the stomach, the bowel, kidneys or allergies. Headaches can be put into two different classifications:

One type of chronic headache can be associated with toxic buildup and illness. A headache is an alarm telling the person that deep down in their body, destruction is going on. Pain and headaches are Mother Nature's great red flashing warning signal to take fast action! There may be trouble anywhere throughout the body. It could be in the liver, gallbladder, kidneys, bowel or any of the body's organs. It may be related to or caused by sensitive sinus, allergy or mucus problems, etc. See pages 54-58 to detox.

Avoid these headache trigger foods:
- Additive and chemical-laced foods
- Salty, sugary or wheat-based foods
- Dairy foods, especially cheese
- Caffeine-containing foods
- Condiments, sulfites, MSG
- Alcohol, beer, wine

– Linda Page, N.D., Ph.D., Author of *Healthy Healing*
See her informative website: *www.healthyhealing.com*

The **second type** of headache is emotional! This is often caused by nervousness, anxiety, stress, strain, tension or any personal or emotional upsets. This is a world where we must be associated with other human beings. Your daily life with others can throw you into many upsetting emotional problems because they can arouse emotions of fear, jealousy, envy, hate, greed, self-pity or self-indulgence. When emotions reach a boiling point, you can usually end up with a dull, throbbing headache. The worst headache is the migraine, which causes the sufferer to feel as if their head is splitting. Do read these three Bragg Books for more health guides:
• *Miracle of Fasting* • *The Bragg Back Fitness Program* and
• *The Bragg Healthy Lifestyle*. See back pages for booklist.

We have found in our many years of research on all kinds of headaches that when the body triggers a headache, the urine is alkaline rather than the normal acid. The kidneys are disturbed by the emotions and it means the body is off-balance. The fast working malic acid of ACV can help relieve headaches by aiding the kidneys to return urine to normal (average 6.4 pH) acidity.

Vaporized ACV can also help relieve headaches. In a vaporizer or small pan, put 2 Tbsps. ACV and 2 cups purified water. Bring mixture to a boil. As vapor begins to rise, turn heat off, put towel over head and lean over steam, taking 5 deep slow breaths of ACV steam vapors. Also for headache relief do some shoulder/neck rolls and massage: head, temples, forehead, sinus areas, neck, shoulders, ears and gently pull lobes, and if needed visit your Chiropractor. For pain use Bromelain 500 mg – it acts like aspirin without the toxic stomach upset. Many chronic headache sufferers have told us they get blessed relief with this method. By doing these things and following The Bragg Healthy Lifestyle, you will have no need for commercial headache remedies and pain killers!

Wise Health Advise from Dean Ornish, M.D. www.ornish.com
We tend to think of advances in medicine as being a new drug, a new surgical technique, a new laser, something high-tech and expensive. We often have a hard time believing that the simple choices that we make each day in our diet and lifestyle can make such a powerful difference in the quality and quantity of our lives, but they most often do. My health program consists of four main components: exercise, nutrition, stress management, love and intimacy and these four promote not only living longer, but living better.

Apple Cider Vinegar for Feet –
Combatting Corns, Callouses and Warts

For Corns and Callouses: First soak affected areas in warm water with ⅓ cup ACV for 20 to 30 minutes. After soaking, rub areas briskly with a coarse towel, then gently use a pumice stone. Now apply a full-strength ACV- soaked gauze bandage overnight, and in the morning prepare a fresh ACV soaked bandage for daytime use. These treatments help soften and dissolve corns and callouses. Check your shoes for comfort and fit. Wrong shoes are the main cause of corns, callouses, bunions and blisters. For casual wear, Birkenstock shoes are great! Give yourself weekly pedicures, massages and exercise your feet daily. Doing this while watching TV is ideal. Treat yourself to foot reflexology therapy (see page 92). Walking barefoot on sand, grass and at home is beneficial. Be good to your feet – they carry you through life! We kept the famous foot doctor going strong and alert for almost 100 years! Dr. Scholl thanked us for our health teachings and said:

"The Bragg *Health Books and Foot Book* are the best!"

For Common Warts: Use the ACV treatment, but caution: *do not rub warts, as this could spread them!* After soaking, use ACV-soaked gauze bandage and keep it on overnight. In the morning, for daytime treatment, apply a castor oil-soaked gauze bandage. At night you can alternate ACV with crushed fresh garlic and vitamin E (prick open capsule). Combination treatments work wonders! If warts become a problem, some doctors freeze them with liquid nitrogen. This method is fast, easy and leaves no scars.

Apple Cider Vinegar Zaps Sore Throat & Laryngitis

Organic, raw ACV is a dangerous enemy to all kinds of germs that attack the throat and mouth! To fight the germs and keep the throat healthy, an ACV gargle mixture works miracles (1 tsp. to ½ glass of water). Gargle 3 mouthfuls of mixture each hour, then spit it out. Don't swallow the gargled mixture, because ACV acts like a sponge, drawing out throat and mouth germs and toxins.

As the throat feels better, gargle every 3 hours. We have famous singers with rock and roll bands, to the Metropolitan Opera's ageless, dynamic 6'6" Jerome Hines to the eternally youthful Beach Boys, using ACV to keep their throats healthy and germ-free. It's important for singers, teachers, ministers, public speakers and you.

Along with the gargling, we use an ACV wet compress as follows: first, place a thin ACV-soaked cloth over throat area, cover with Saran Wrap, then use a flat hot water bottle or moist, hot wrung-out towel to heat the area, allowing ACV to absorb through the skin. This ACV hot compress is also great for cleansing and healing the chest area when treating all lung congestions – colds, flu, bronchitis, emphysema and asthma. It feels good, too.

Even in good health, use ACV gargle twice weekly to remove any body toxins being eliminated through the throat tissues. The gargle is also helpful during fasting, when the throat may produce a stringy mucus as part of the detoxifying process! Read our *Miracle of Fasting* book: it contains the powerful health message of fasting to detox, cleanse and renew the body. See pages 54 to 58.

Apple Cider Vinegar for Healthy Skin

Reap vitality with the apple cider vinegar massage: To a small basin of warm water, add ½ cup of ACV. Dip both hands in mixture and massage this all over your body (in shower or bathtub): face, neck, chest, arms, shoulders, back, abdomen, legs and feet. Massage mixture into skin thoroughly and be gentle on the face. This leaves skin soft and pH balanced. Healthy skin has an acid reaction, for it is throwing off toxic poisons through its billions of pores. (Skin is often called your third kidney.)

After thoroughly wetting the skin with the mixture several times, rub and massage until the skin is dry. Do this at least twice a week and do not wash it off; leave it on the body. As you massage the mixture into the skin, you will feel a new vitality coming into your body.

Don't Recycle Body Mucus!
Your body's machinery works hard to collect the mucus in your body and then push it out your nose or mouth. So, when it's ready to get out – spit – cough – blow it out! Please – never recycle mucus by swallowing it!

The reason this treatment is far better than using soap is because soap has an alkaline reaction on the skin and you don't want that! By keeping the skin in an acid reaction, it will help you have healthier skin. I've never used soap on my face or body, just ACV and it's worked wonders. If you want to use soap – Castile soap is best.

We find after hard exercise or long mental work that we get a new feeling of strength and energy after one of these ACV massages. Also try gentle dry skin brushing with loofah pad or vegetable brush next time you feel mentally or physically tired. It helps remove old skin cells and toxic wastes. We know you'll want to do it often. The health benefits of improved circulation are obvious!

Apple Cider Vinegar for Skin Problems

To open the pores and loosen dirt and grease from your face, turn off heat under a pan of steaming ACV water (3 Tbsp. ACV to a quart of purified water). Steam face over pan and use towel draped over head to trap steam. Then pat ACV on face with cotton ball to remove loosened dirt. Repeat steaming and cleansing twice. Then you can gently squeeze out any blackheads. Then pat or spray on chilled ACV, diluted with equal amount of distilled water (store ACV mixture in refrigerator) to close pores and tone skin. Do steam cleansing twice weekly, as needed. Another excellent cleanser and toner is aloe gel or fresh aloe vera cactus pulp. Cut off 1 inch of aloe vera rib, slit open and rub yellowish pulp directly on the skin. We grow our own aloe plants – you can grow them in pots also. Aloe is a great healer for burns, pimples, sores, bites, etc!

Apple Cider Vinegar for Sunburns

Gently pat undiluted ACV on skin to give relief from sunburn. Leave it on to help prevent blistering and peeling. For all-over sunburns, pour 1 cup of ACV in cool bath water, then enjoy the healing soak. After soaking, gently dry body, then pat ACV directly to needed areas. Wait 5 minutes, then pat on aloe vera gel. We receive many wonderful ACV testimonials. See one on page 35.

Younger Looking Skin in Minutes With Apple Cider Vinegar Facial

The skin consists of microscopically small, flat scales that constantly flake off, thereby revealing the new skin beneath the outer, older layer of scales. In millions of people, the old, tired, dead, dry outer scales do not peel off promptly, slowing new growth and leaving their skin dry, sallow, dull and lifeless. This is known as "the old-age look".

Men and women can use this ACV facial for amazing results! First, wash skin in warm water (no soap). Next, apply a wrung-out, hot water-soaked cloth to the face for 3 minutes, then remove. Soak thin cloth in warm ACV water (1 Tbsp. ACV per cup of water) and again apply to face. Cover ACV-soaked cloth with a towel wrung out in hot water. Now lie down for 10 minutes or longer with your feet elevated on couch, against wall, or use a slant board or an ironing board. This brings more blood circulation to the face for cell rejuvenation.

Remove both cloths and gently rub skin upwards with a coarse towel or our favorite – a small loofah face pad. This rub removes the hundreds of old, dry skin scales that have been detached and loosened by the ACV facial. You can repeat this weekly or as needed. Your skin will look more youthful and will shine like a polished apple with joyous new life. We should all have pride in looking our best and presenting a good personal appearance. You will be truly amazed and proud of yourself with the results from these age-reversing, simple health treatments!

We must always change, renew, rejuvenate ourselves; otherwise, we harden. – Johann W. Goethe

Sad Facts: Many people go throughout life committing partial suicide – destroying their health, skin, heart, youth, beauty, talents, energies and creative qualities. Indeed, to learn how to be good to oneself is often more difficult than to learn how to be good to others. – Paul C. Bragg

Prayer is the mortar that holds our house together. – Sister Teresa, James 5:16

Love is the cement that binds families together, but it is friendship that makes them happy. – William Hazlitt

Skin Problems and Treatments

ACV can be used to effectively relieve the pain and discomfort of **cold sores and genital sores** caused by the herpes virus. Apply ACV directly to the affected areas and the itching and burning discomfort will rapidly dissipate. ACV also helps the sores to heal more quickly.

Shingles and chicken pox, caused by herpes zoster virus, can be relieved with straight ACV applications. Gently apply to the itching and burning areas. A cup of ACV in a warm bath will also help soothe itching.

ACV relieves the itching and discomfort caused by **poison ivy and poison oak** and other poisonous plants. Mix equal parts of ACV and distilled water and spray on the affected areas to stop the pain, itching and ease the redness and swelling. Keep spray mixture in refrigerator; a cold spray is more soothing. (Read bottom of * page 25.)

Healing is faster for **minor cuts and abrasions**, and there is less chance of infection if you swab areas with ACV (perfect disinfectant and healer) daily. ACV also helps stop bleeding by helping the blood to clot. Soak a cotton ball in ACV and press on abrasion until bleeding stops.

Varicose veins can be unsightly and painful, but applications of ACV can help shrink the veins. Wrap an ACV-dampened cloth around needed areas both morning and night, then elevate legs, leaving on for 15 minutes (follow instructions on page 23). Then remove wrap, legs still up – start at ankles to gently press over pooled veins to get blood back into circulation. To help speed up the inner cleansing and healing, remember to drink and enjoy your Bragg ACV cocktail 3 times daily.

Relief from **dry, itchy skin and hives** will come after applying a paste of ACV and cornstarch to affected areas. The ACV paste mixture draws out the itching as it dries.

Oily skin can be helped by the ACV drink and the facial treatment twice a week, explained on page 23.

To help prevent **windburn, sunburn and chapping** coat the exposed skin with a 50/50 ACV and Bragg Organic Olive Oil mixture. When in the elements, carry this mixture along.

ACV For Insect Stings, Bites, Ear Infections, Yeast and Fungus Problems

ACV helps stop pain and itching from **mosquito** and other **insect bites, bee stings** and also it neutralizes the **jellyfish's painful venom**. Use straight ACV on affected areas or an ACV compress as often as needed. ACV also helps **middle ear infections** and **swimmer's ear,** a condition from swimming and showering, which may cause temporary loss of hearing. Dilute ACV with equal parts distilled water and drop into ear for ear infections, ear aches and if you feel a blockage in your ears. Drug stores stock ear dropper syringes. If ear problems persist, see a health professional.

For **hemorrhoids and rectal itching**, soak cotton ball in ACV and gently press on area for immediate relief.

Yeast and fungus infections of the body and mucus membranes (such as **thrush** in the mouth and throat, on genital areas on males and females – especially children – such as **diaper rash** and **jock itch, athlete's foot** and **eczema**) can all be treated with a 50/50 solution of ACV and distilled water. For athlete's foot, soak feet in 50/50 mixture of ACV and lukewarm water twice daily; for mouth thrush, gargle every 3 hours with 1 tsp. ACV in half glass of warm water. Also slowly drink a warm Bragg ACV cocktail morning and night. For genital areas, especially in the case of itch or diaper rash* on infants, swab affected area carefully with a solution of 1 Tbsps. ACV to 1 quart warm distilled water 3 times daily. The treatments for all yeast infections should continue for at least 10 days or until symptoms dissipate.

The true doctor will be a teacher; his work will be to keep them well, instead of trying to heal them after sickness. – Ralph W. Trine

---

Fixing Life's Flats: When your life seems a bit flat, look around for a source of leakage! Life habits, actions, words, deeds, thoughts - are they healthy and happy? Just a little leak will in time cause a tire to go flat, also your life! Check your life for leaks and stop them now! – Patricia Bragg

---

* *If it persists, try aloe vera or calendula, comfrey or MSM ointments for healing of rashes on humans – babies, children, adults – even animals.*

Apple Cider Vinegar for Dandruff, Itching Scalp, Dry and Thinning Hair and Baldness

The high acidity (organic malic acid) plus the powerful enzymes (the "mother's" life chemicals) in ACV kill the bottle bacillus, a germ responsible for many scalp and hair conditions. The problems caused by this are dandruff, itching scalp, thinning hair and often baldness.

Every hair has its own oil can. Bottle bacilli can clog these tiny openings. Scales and small dry crusts are formed, resulting in itching and dandruff. The oil-starved hairs either fall out or break off, causing thinning of the hair and often baldness. ACV not only kills bottle bacillus, but stimulates the oil cans to a healthier, more balanced activity.

Pour 3 Tbsps. ACV in cup – part the hair in sections and sponge ACV directly onto scalp and wrap head with a towel. For dry hair weekly apply castor oil or olive oil to hair, and ACV to scalp, then wrap. Leave on for 30 minutes to 3 hours before shampooing. The ACV helps restore the proper acid/alkaline balance to scalp. For acute cases, do daily or before every shampoo. **Hair growth stimulating mixture:** for bald and thinning areas – pat this mixture on scalp (2 Tbsp ACV and ¼ tsp cayenne powder), hour before shampooing (keep out of eyes!). Many get great results.

Hair rinse mixture: for a healthy after-shampoo rinse for shine and body. add ⅓ cup ACV to quart of water. Pre-mix in plastic bottle and keep in shower to use.

For Muscle Soreness and Aching Joints

To soothe tired, aching muscles and joints, there is nothing like an ACV bath combined with a self-massage. While soaking in a warm bath with 1 cup ACV added, massage entire body, starting at feet. Gently squeeze and relax each part of the foot, working slowly up right leg to hip, then left leg. Continue up torso, arms and neck, always rubbing toward the heart. For the face, lightly stroke skin in upward direction; avoid pulling facial skin down. Finish with firm fingertip dry massage in circular motions over the scalp, then finger rub your ears.

For pain and stiffness, arthritis, osteoarthritis and to help heal and regenerate cartilage and bones use glucosamine and chrondroitin sulfates and MSM combo – works miracles!

For Arrhythmia and Strengthening Heart

Enjoy your basic 3 Bragg ACV cocktails daily! Plus have another ½ tsp. ACV in ½ glass of distilled water, twice daily between meals, ideal before brisk walk or exercise.

The heart, a large muscle and your master pump uses large amounts of potassium to keep going strong for your entire life! It's the hardest working muscle in the body (see page 6). It must have a constant, continuous supply of power and energy to continue beating. ACV contains a natural chemical that combines with heart fuel to make the heart muscle stronger and helps normalize blood pressure and cholesterol. To help arrhythmia also take Magnesium, CoQ10, Folic Acid, B6 and B12 supplements.

Low Fat Meals Cut Heart Disease Risk

A great British research report by Dr. George Miller of Britain's Medical Research Council stated: *"High fat meals make the blood more prone to clot within 6 to 7 hours after eating. Low fat meals can almost immediately reverse this condition. Most heart attacks occur in the early morning. One reason may be the overnight clotting effects of a high fat dinner. Researchers feel that by cutting fats from your diet, you may be able to add years to your life and cut the risk of heart disease!"* University of Chicago and Stanford's research supports Dr. Miller's statement that the healthy heart, low fat vegetarian meals with ample fresh fruits and vegetables are the best and safest. (See Healthy Heart Habits page 87.)

How to Improve the Digestion

Millions suffer with indigestion, which is aggravated by poor digestion and weak saliva juices. This causes distress: gas, heartburn, burping and stomach bloating. Before mealtime, sip ⅓ tsp. Bragg ACV. Hold in mouth for a minute before swallowing. This promotes enzymes and saliva, which helps the digestion that starts in the mouth. This causes stomach digestive fluids to flow faster, resulting in improved digestion and better health.

Bragg Organic Apple Cider Vinegar with the "mother" is vital to the body's digestive balance by stimulating the flow of precious enzymes and saliva in the mouth. I recommend to stop heartburn and indigestion and also to improve digestion, sip ⅓ teaspoon ACV before meals to activate the flow of digestive juices. – Gabriel Cousens, M.D., Author, Conscious Eating

Chewing Gum Habit Causes Stomach Problems

Please never chew gum because it fools the body into thinking food is coming and causes precious digestive juices to start flowing. These powerful juices can cause trouble with your empty stomach's lining, resulting in ulcers, stomach problems, heartburn, bloating, gas, etc.

Fight Kidney and Bladder Problems

Avoid all animal, dairy, salt, alcohol and sugar products. All ages should follow The Bragg Healthy Lifestyle for health. Use ACV on salads and have your ACV drink 3 times daily. ACV can help bladder problems and dissolve some types of stones. Drink 8 glasses of distilled water, plus some organic, unsweetened cranberry juice. Add ⅓ tsp. ACV to each glass, which helps acidify urine, inhibits bacterial growth and promotes healing. You may sweeten the cranberry drink with organic grape juice or raw honey. You can also do a 2 or 3 day watermelon only flush. Thoroughly chew and swallow the seeds, too. This is a great kidney – bladder cleanser and healer.

For bedwetting: Mix ½ to 1 tsp. buckwheat honey with ½ tsp. ACV before bedtime. It's also best to stop liquids 3 hours before bedtime, except for small sips.

For all kidney and bladder problems: Children and adults should drink 8 glasses daily of distilled water. It's important for the urinary tract and kidneys. Use this healing and cleansing drink: 2 Tbsp *fresh or dried corn silk to 1 quart distilled water or try marshmallow herbal tea, 2 to 3 times daily. Add ½ tsp. ACV to each cup and sweeten with 1 tsp. buckwheat honey. (* Save and dry corn silks from fresh corn and store in an airtight bottle.)

To soothe and heal bladder infections: Add 1 cup ACV to warm low sitz bath. Use 1 to 2 times daily. Also, ACV douches help (page 30). Use a dipstick tester from the drugstore to check for any urinary infection.*

To eliminate "dribbles": To keep the bladder and sphincter muscles tightened and toned – urinate – stop – urinate – stop, 6 times, twice daily when voiding. This simple exercise works. After age 40, do this every day.

---

*Important: We don't endorse antibiotics, but if you ever take them, please take acidophilus liquid or capsules to replace the friendly bacteria in your body.

Apple Cider Vinegar Combats Gallstones

Before starting the 2 day gallbladder flush, prepare for 1 week by drinking slowly – upon arising, at mid-morning, mid-afternoon and after dinner – ½ tsp ACV with a 6 ounce glass of apple juice; or if hypoglycemic or diabetic, dilute with half distilled water. Organic, unfiltered apple juice is rich in malic acid, potassium, pectins and enzymes. These act as solvents to soften and help remove debris (small stones, etc.) and cleanse the body. Doctors have non-surgical methods for removing the difficult, larger stones using sound waves. But it's best to purge small and medium-sized ones twice yearly. These are the ones that can grow to cause problems!

No food is eaten (only liquids) during the following 2 day gallbladder flush. Combine in 8 oz glass: ⅓ Bragg Organic Olive Oil (no substitutes), ⅔ apple juice (organic) and 1 tsp. Bragg Organic ACV. Drink this mixture 3 times the first day. *At night, sleep on your right side when on flush, pulling right knee toward chest to open pathway.* On the second day, take mixture twice. On both days drink all apple juice desired, but no water or any other liquid. This is not for diabetics unless supervised by a health professional.

About midmorning on the third day, eat a raw variety salad (nature's broom) of cabbage, carrots, celery, beets, tomatoes, sprouts and lettuce, with lots of ACV and olive oil. If desired, have a bowl of lightly steamed greens, such as kale, collards, chard or other leafy greens. Season with ACV, olive oil, brewer's yeast flakes and a spray of Bragg Aminos – this gives delicious flavor to all greens.

We take this miracle cleanser flush at least once or twice a year. Check your bowel movements for tiny, greenish-brown stones. It will amaze you what your gallbladder, stomach and colon will flush out!

Distilled water plays vital part in treatment of illness, arthritis, etc. – Dr. Banik

Everyone should be his own physician.
We ought to assist and not force nature. – Voltaire

Nature, time and patience are the three great physicians. – Irish Proverb

Happiness is not being pained in body or troubled in mind.
– Thomas Jefferson, Third U.S. President

Note: Some nausea may occur. This shows toxins, mucus and bile are being dumped in the stomach. Your body wants it out! If nauseated, your body is saying: "Drink 1 to 2 glasses of distilled water and regurgitate until stomach is empty." (You might have to depress your tongue while leaning over the bowl.) Once it's out, you will feel better right away! Remember, it's always the wisest decision when you are nauseated to get out whatever is causing an upset stomach!

Apple Cider Vinegar Helps Shrink Prostate

With a fork, "whip" 2 Tbsps. ACV with 2 Tbsps. Bragg Organic Olive Oil, a dash of Bragg Liquid Aminos and cinnamon. Use this ACV mixture daily over salads, sliced tomatoes, avocados and steamed veggies. Enjoy with meals, zinc-rich raw pumpkin seeds. Zinc, Prostex and Saw Palmetto supplements are healing for prostate.

Apple Cider Vinegar for Female Troubles

For a healthier vagina, use ACV douches and baths when needed, as ACV acidity is the same as the vagina's.

Douche mixture: 3 Tbsps. ACV to 2 quarts warm distilled water is a cleansing, healing douche. If discharge is present, use 1 to 2 times daily, but less frequently as discharge lessens. **For bath:** Add 2 cups ACV to water.

To shrink, tighten and tone a flabby womb, eat raw garden salads made with extra parsley and celery. Sprinkle salads with ACV, Bragg Olive Oil and a spray of Bragg Liquid Aminos over the top. Also exercise daily!

Fight Arthritis with Apple Cider Vinegar

Hard, stony deposits fill up, cement, enlarge and cripple the joints! Crippling, painful arthritis and joint problems are the sad result! Flush out those stony deposits with your daily ACV drinks. Upon arising, an hour before lunch and dinner have your delicious ACV cocktail as follows: Stir 8 ounces distilled water with 1 to 2 tsps. equally of ACV and raw honey (diabetics use stevia). Also add ACV to your salads and steamed greens. Be faithful to The Bragg Healthy Lifestyle and your 24 hour fasts. Eat 60% to 70% healthy, raw foods (organic is best) and drink

8 glasses daily of distilled water (free of chemicals and inorganic mineral). To heal and regenerate, take natural multi-vitamin-minerals, Glucosamine, Chondroitin Sulfates and MSM combo supplements, plus alfalfa tablets and 1 to 2 tsps. of cod liver oil daily. Improvements are amazing, plus enjoy 2 organic apples a day to help keep the doctor away!

Apple Cider Vinegar Combats Mucus

Millions have postnasal drip and are plagued with toxic mucus in their sinus cavities, nose and throat, which is most uncomfortable! If mucus sufferers remove all dairy products, eggs and sugars from their diet, follow The Bragg Healthy Lifestyle, take a weekly 24-hour fast and use ample ACV, soon these mucus conditions will vanish on this healthy toxicless and mucusless diet!

Upon arising, have glass of warm distilled water with 1 – 2 tsps. ACV and 1 – 2 tsps. raw honey (recipe pg 96). Also enjoy this drink midmorning and mid-afternoon. On your salads use 1 to 2 tsps. ACV combined with Bragg Olive Oil and a dash or spray of Bragg Liquid Aminos. Try our delicious, all-purpose Bragg Aminos in the handy, small spray bottle. This is a great method for seasoning salads, potatoes, vegetables, etc., and even popcorn! The spray bottle is perfect to take along when dining out!

For throat gargle and nasal wash: Add 1-2 tsps. ACV to ½ glass warm water for throat gargle (page 20) or nasal sniff wash to help clean out the mucus. Sniff up right nostril, roll head back, then side to side, lean over, blow out mucus. Then repeat with other side. Do 2x daily until mucus conditions subside. Along with the ACV drink, enjoy fresh carrot and green juices between meals. It's important to sip and savor fresh juices slowly, as they are really foods, not just beverages. Small amounts of juice (or food) in the mouth at one time will be better digested and more easily used by the body chemistry.

ACV mouthwash: (tsp ACV to ½ glass water) Kills mouth bacteria, fights plaque and tartar, helps prevent gum disease (page 38), promotes healing and freshens breath.

At mealtime come thou hither and eat of the bread and dip the morsel in the vinegar. – Ruth 2:14

For Nosebleeds

Soak a cotton ball or gauze in ACV and lightly pack in nostrils. Relax, sit down and lean forward for 10 minutes (breathe through mouth) pressing nostrils together while ACV pack helps blood congeal. Repeat if needed. Vitamins C and K are helpful. Be sure to drink 8 glasses of distilled water daily – nosebleeds are often caused by dehydration.

Apple Cider Vinegar and Constipation

It's important that the bowels move regularly and freely. Outgo should equal intake. You should have a bowel movement soon after arising and within an hour after meals. Flaxseeds and its' tea with ACV act as bowel lubricants, as do fresh fruits, vegetables and distilled water.

Make the ACV-Flaxseed Bowel Lubricant Mixture: Boil two cups distilled water with 4 Tbsps. flaxseeds for 15 minutes or soak overnight. Mixture becomes jellylike when cold. Stir 2 Tbsps. of mixture, plus 1 tsp. ACV in glass of distilled water (add blackstrap molasses or honey if desired sweetened). Drink upon arising and an hour before bed. Store mixture in refrigerator and use when needed.

Use Miracle Psyllium Husk Powder For Healthy Elimination: Add 1 Tbsp. of this super cleansing herb to any of these: Bragg ACV drink, juice, glass distilled water, herb tea, cereals, soups, etc.; let it soak two minutes before drinking or eating! This helps cleanse the mucus along the small intestine and colon walls and pulls toxins from the gastrointestinal tract. Also use Bragg Organic Olive Oil over salads, veggies, potatoes, etc. – it helps elimination and detoxifies the colon, plus adds delicious flavor to foods.

To check bowel elimination time: Have some fresh or frozen whole corn with your evening meal. Purposely don't chew all the kernels. (Always chew food thoroughly otherwise.) Check your stools to see when the corn is eliminated, usually within 14 hours. When it's cleansed of toxins and malnutrition is treated, the body becomes healthier and starts working more normally. Because constipation brings on many health problems, including arthritis, it's important to keep the pipes (colon and arteries) clean and open by following The Bragg Healthy Lifestyle.

It's natural to squat to have bowel movements. It opens up anal area more directly. When on toilet, putting feet up 6 to 8 inches on waste basket or footstool gives the same squatting effect. Now raise and stretch your hands above your head so that the transverse colon can empty completely with ease. It's important to drink 8 glasses of pure water daily! (Read page 87 and take your psyllium husk powder daily.)

The body is 70% water and pure, steam-distilled (chemical-free) water is important for total health. You should drink at least 8 glasses of water daily. Read our book, *Water – The Shocking Truth*, for more info on the importance of pure water. See back pages for booklist.

What Becomes of the Acid Crystals Precipitated in the Body That Age Us?

You have often heard the expression, "He's stiff and old and his flesh is tough." When you think of "old" people you usually think of them as having stiffness in their body, with tough, brittle flesh (see Dr. Carrel's study on page 10). Why do people get stiff in the joints and their flesh tough when they have added birthdays to their life? Most people would answer this complex question with the remark, "Because they are old". But this isn't the real answer why people get stiff joints and tough flesh. The answer to premature ageing is unhealthy living and potassium deficiency! People rarely study their bodies or learn what to eat for healthy tissues and youthful joints (ACV brings miracles). They are satisfied to eat what agrees with them. Or they eat foods they were reared on as children and carry these early eating habits (often unhealthy) right into their adult life and then into their children's lives!

WATER IS KEY TO HEALTH & ALL BODY FUNCTIONS:		
• Elimination	• Muscles	• Nerves
• Circulation	• Metabolism	• Energy
• Digestion	• Assimilation	• Sex
• Bones & Joints	• Heart	• Glands

Rearing Healthy Children is Important

The Bragg family children, grandchildren and great-grandchildren have all been reared on The Bragg Healthy Lifestyle. We were taught to keep in perfect health so that the body tissues would remain soft and tender and have elasticity and health. This correct way of eating enables us to come to the later years of life with youthful looking skin, keen hearing, sharp, sparkling eyes and perfect mental, emotional and physical health, for a long, useful, happy and healthy life.

Miracles with Apple Cider Vinegar

The members of the Bragg family follow The Bragg Healthy Lifestyle. They have learned the lessons of good nutrition and the miracles of ACV for themselves and their animals. The children were impressed when Farmer Bragg would have an old hen prepared for dinner. The old hen's meat was tough and didn't taste good. This is what happens to poultry and beef when it is deficient in potassium. Human flesh suffers the same problems.

To prove to the children conclusively that apple cider vinegar and honey needed to be an important part of their daily nutrition, he would then select another old hen for the dinner table. This time he fed that old hen ACV twice a day, for ten days. When the hen was prepared for the dinner table, the children tasted the difference in the old hen's meat. They noticed how tender it was – just like a young hen and they asked for second helpings. (P.S. Most of the Bragg family members are now happy, thriving, heart-healthy vegetarians!)

Miracles can happen everyday – through guidance and prayer!

True prayer is not only experienced in words, it emanates through your entire being in the form of your thoughts as well as actions. – Amrit Desai

Children are very responsive to healthy lifestyle changes, and those start with providing the right foods (fruits, vegetables, whole grains and reasonable amounts of other healthful snacks), encouraging regular exercise and activity and limiting television, video and web watching!
– Susan K. Rhodes, Ph.D., Medical University of South Carolina

A friend may well be reckoned the masterpiece of nature.
– Ralph Waldo Emerson

"Apple Cider Vinegar Cures Burns"

Here's a testimonial from Joel & N'omi Orr, Chesapeake, VA:
We have used Bragg's Apple Cider Vinegar for several years and love your wonderful book about it. We want to share with you something that we believe is one of the greatest benefits Bragg's Organic Apple Cider Vinegar brings to humanity (commercial vinegars don't have the same effect): Bragg's Apple Cider Vinegar, if splashed on a burn of any kind, stops the intense, continual pain instantly and permanently! It also prevents scarring! We not only keep a bottle in our kitchen, we also keep bottles in our cars to use when people get burned from hot engines, radiators, etc. When traveling, we have helped burn victims from accidents in restaurant kitchens, cars, etc. We suggest everyone keep a bottle of Bragg's Vinegar nearby! Everyone who has tried it, has praised it. Bragg's Vinegar is the best burn healer in the world, no matter how bad the burn! We thank you! The Orrs

The Miracle Life of Jack LaLanne

Jack LaLanne, Patricia Bragg, Elaine LaLanne & Paul C. Bragg

Jack says he would have been dead by 16 if he hadn't attended The Bragg Crusade. Jack says, *Bragg saved my life at age 15, when I attended the Bragg Health and Fitness Crusade in Oakland, California.* From that day, Jack has continued to live The Bragg Healthy Lifestyle, inspiring millions to health, fitness and a long and happy life!

See web: www.jacklalanne.com

Create the highest, grandest vision for your life, because you become what you believe." – Oprah Winfrey

All Through Life You Fight Acid Crystals

When acid crystals harden in the joints and tissues, the joints become stiff and the tissues hardened. The meat becomes tough and tasteless. When the animals are given apple cider vinegar regularly, the precipitated acid crystals enter into a solution and pass out of the body, thus making the body tissues healthier and tender. This applies to human flesh also. Now, when body tissues hold all the precipitated acid crystals they can, the crystals then appear in the bursae and the joints of the body, resulting in bursitis and arthritis. 1 to 2 tsps. of apple cider vinegar with 1 to 2 tsps. of raw honey in a glass of distilled water 3 times daily will help relieve stiff, aching, prematurely old joints. You be the judge. See how elastic and flexible all your joints become!

Keep Your Joints and Tissues Youthful

Most people have lost their normal contact with Mother Nature and simple, natural living. They no longer know how to eat the simple way God intended. If you suffer from prematurely old joints and hardened tissues, be sure to take the ACV mixture three times daily. Eliminate or cut down on animal proteins. Stop all refined sugars, products and beverages! Then you will see how very youthful your body begins to feel.

Toxic Acid Arthritic Crystals Make Joints Grind

The grinding sound you hear in your neck when you roll your head is the toxic arthritic acid crystals that have deposited themselves on the uppermost bone of your spine – the Atlas. Just as ACV washes sludge off windows, it also washes the body sludge from the joints and cardiovascular system of the body. Fasting, and taking the Bragg's Apple Cider Vinegar Cocktail will help eliminate the acid crystals from the joints. A feeling of agelessness gradually will replace that tight, stiff, ageing feeling. You will start to feel more flexible, pain-free and loose in every moveable joint of your body.

Loving thoughts are little seeds . . . Let them blossom into deeds.

Roses and flowers are God's autograph.

ACV Helps Stiffness Vanish From Body

You will find, after several months of the ACV and honey cocktail taken 3 times daily – that the stiffness and misery will be gone from your joints and body. You will discover you can walk or run up several flights of stairs without any effort and pain. Also follow page 87. You will notice that you look, act and feel younger!

Make The Bragg Healthy Lifestyle a life-long daily habit! Over the years we have seen many stiff-jointed, prematurely old people transform themselves into new, youthful, healthy people! We can't do it for you. You must make the effort to give this ACV and Bragg Healthy Lifestyle a chance to prove what it can do for you!

Questions About Apple Cider Vinegar

Many people have some preconceived idea that apple cider vinegar is harmful to the body. Instead it's the distilled, pasteurized, filtered, the malt and synthetic, dead vinegars that must be avoided for human consumption!

Let us assure you that there is nothing in this wonderful, organic, raw ACV that can in any way harm your body! People ask us about the merits and benefits of ACV. See the inside front cover for a list of some of the miracles it can perform and has for centuries.

Animal proteins and fats have a tendency to thicken the blood, while the natural acids and enzymes in ACV help to keep the blood healthier and thinner. Also, that's why people naturally crave and serve cranberry sauce, which contains four different natural acids, with turkey and other fowl. They serve applesauce with roast pork dishes and a slice of lemon with fish, or steak with mushrooms, all rich in natural acids.

Works and deeds, not words, are the proof of love!

The use of organic apple cider vinegar is a wonderful health aid, and the #1 food I recommend in helping to maintain the body's vital acid-alkaline balance. Everyone should read this Bragg Apple Cider Vinegar *book.*
– Gabriel Cousens, M.D., Author of *Conscious Eating* and *Spiritual Nutrition*

ACV Helps Normalize Blood Pressure

Natural food acids served along with animal proteins are designed to lessen the blood thickening influence of these heavy proteins. In order for blood to circulate freely throughout the body, it must be thin. When blood thickens, it strains the heart. The blood pressure then goes up and a host of other health problems begin.

Remember, blood has to circulate all over the body through the arteries, blood vessels and tiny capillaries. It's impossible for blood to circulate freely through these hair-like pipes when it is thickened with too many heavy protein meals, fats, hardened oils, etc.

Several years ago, we met a woman with extremely high blood pressure. We put her on a two day ACV, honey and water fast program with nothing to eat for 48 hours. She had an ACV cocktail 5 times daily, plus 5 glasses of pure distilled water – total of 10 glasses.

In 48 hours, her blood pressure had dropped to almost normal! The buzzing in her ears ceased, and her dull headache stopped. After a short period of correct eating (no salt, sugar, saturated fats, tea, coffee, etc.) combined with The Bragg Healthy Lifestyle and ACV program her blood pressure was normal and she felt reborn!

People ask us if ACV will make them slender. It helps balance the body chemistry and normalize the body weight. We have been using the ACV program in the Bragg family for over five generations and it has brought wonderful results for our health and our trim bodies.

Evidence reveals that ACV has been shown to lower blood pressure and strengthen the heart muscle because it acts as a blood thinner and reduces the risk of a stroke. It contains important potassium which is also vital and needed to keep the heart and bloodstream healthy.

Everything is brighter in the new dawn's light –
especially after a recharging, good night's sleep!

The more natural food you eat, the more radiant health you will enjoy and you will be better able to promote the higher life of love and brotherhood. – Patricia Bragg

Studies show low CoQ10 levels cause heart disease, declining memory and brain function and periodontal conditions.
– Dr. Stephen Sinatra, Coenzyme Q10 Phemomenon www.sinatramd.com

The Bragg Healthy Lifestyle Promotes Super Health

The Bragg Healthy Lifestyle consists of eating 60%-70% fresh, organic, live foods: raw vegetables, salads, sprouts, fresh fruits and fresh juices; raw seeds and nuts; 100% whole grain breads, pastas, cereals, nutritious beans and legumes. These are the good (no cholesterol, no fat, no salt, no sugar) "live foods" – the body fuel required for lively, healthy people! This is the reason people become revitalized and reborn into a fresh, new life filled with joy, health, vitality, youthfulness and longevity! There are millions of Bragg Healthy Lifestyle followers around the world! When it works for you, please write and share your results with us, we love hearing from our book friends!

Five Generations of Healthy Braggs Give Thanks to Using Apple Cider Vinegar

Since birth, all the Bragg children have used ACV. They fed it to their children and now their grandchildren are feeding it to the great-grandchildren! We all use ACV along with Bragg Organic Olive Oil on our salads. We put both on our steamed greens (cabbage, chard, collards, kale, spinach, mustard and beet greens, broccoli, Brussels sprouts and cauliflower) and use with many other foods.

Millions of our students around the world have used ACV and never once has anyone reported a negative reaction from using it. In fact, they sing its praises! So, you also will soon see the benefits from using Bragg ACV and following The Bragg Healthy Lifestyle Program.

"All vinegar is not created equal. Bragg Organic Apple Cider Vinegar is made from fresh, crushed organic apples and then matured in wooden barrels. It's smoother and so much healthier than other vinegars. Apple cider vinegar is healthful because it's loaded with vitamins, minerals and rich in potassium. Apple Cider Vinegar helps balance the body's vital acid/alkaline balance. . . . *Do As I Do – Drink the Bragg's Apple Vinegar Drink daily!* "
– Julian Whitaker, M.D., *Health and Healing Newsletter* www.drwhitaker.com

The body and the mind are so closely connected that not even a single word or thought can come into existence without being reflected in the personality and health of the individual. – John Prentiss

Apple Cider Vinegar and Arthritis

People ask if ACV cures arthritis. This is not possible, for curing is an internal biological function that only the body can perform. We have seen miracles how ACV fights arthritis, along with a healthy diet, exercise, deep breathing, rest, relaxation and living The Bragg Healthy Lifestyle are required to put the body in a condition to cure itself. ACV is an important part of the program (page 30). When all Mother Nature's supreme forces are used, the body will turn from sickness to wellness. Health is something you must desire, seek out, earn and always guard and treasure for your life's sake!

Apple Cider Vinegar Relieves Muscle Cramps

Many people are awakened in the middle of the night with sharp, painful muscle cramps. These often occur in the feet and lower or upper legs. Sometimes they occur in the stomach, intestines and occasionally in the heart. These are frightening experiences! Most people who experience leg cramps are forced to jump out of bed and pound or firmly massage the area to get relief. Many people with cramps in other parts of the body have to walk quickly to get relief. When precipitated acid crystals get into the circulation of the legs and other parts of the body, they can cause severe cramps. We recommend taking 2 tsps. ACV and 2 tsps. of honey in a glass of distilled water three times daily to relieve these painful cramps. This allows the precipitated acid crystals to enter into a solution and pass out of the body, causing cramps to cease. Calcium and also magnesium orotate supplements taken before bedtime can also help prevent cramping, plus they promote sound sleep.

Acid Crystals Cause Premature Ageing

Everyone, even the healthiest person in the world, must continually fight the buildup of acid crystals in the body. The strongest enemy of acid crystals is the organic apple cider vinegar, raw honey and distilled water cocktail. This powerful mixture puts the acid crystals in solution so they can be flushed out of the body by the kidneys and other organs of elimination.

Take This 48 Hour Test

For 2 full days, take nothing into your system but liquids. Have the ACV cocktail 3 to 5 times daily, plus another 4 to 5 glasses of distilled water daily as well. Ample water is needed to flush the toxins out!

On the second and third day, after you have eaten nothing else for 48 hours, take a sample of your first morning urine and store in labeled bottles with tight lids. Keep on shelf for 2 weeks, then examine sediment at bottom of bottles. These are some of the disease-causing toxins that were flushed out of your body!

Potassium – The Master Mineral

Always keep in mind the fact that potassium puts toxic poisons in solution so they can be flushed out of the body. **The body is self-cleansing, self-correcting, self-repairing and self-healing!** Just give it the tools to work with and soon you can enjoy a painless, tireless, ageless body, regardless of age! Forget age and calendar years, for age isn't toxic! You age prematurely when you suffer from malnutrition and potassium deficiencies. These cause low Vital Force and waste buildups and poor elimination that causes disease to proliferate.

The Bragg Healthy Lifestyle will help you rebuild your Vital Force. Watch the transformation that will take place in your body when you faithfully follow your ACV regimen. You can and will create the kind of person you want to be! Plan, plot and follow through! Start now!

Although you must follow this program closely, please don't try to do everything listed immediately. Remember, it took you a long time of living by wrong habits to cause any of the problems your body might have now. So, it's going to take time for the body to cleanse, repair and rebuild itself into a more *perfect healthy home* for you! Please remember, your body is your temple while on this earth, so cherish it and protect it!

Many studies have shown that people who lower their blood cholesterol levels by diet can slow, or even reverse atherosclerosis and cut risk of having a heart attack. –University of California, Berkeley *Wellness Letter* www.berkleywellness.com

WE THANK THEE

For flowers that bloom about our feet;
   For song of bird and hum of bee;
For all things fair we hear or see,
   Father in heaven we thank Thee!
For blue of stream and blue of sky;
   For pleasant shade of branches high;
For fragrant air and cooling breeze;
   For beauty of the blooming trees;
Father in heaven we thank Thee!
   For mother love and father care,
For brothers strong and sisters fair;
   For love at home and here each day;
For guidance lest we go astray,
   Father in heaven we thank Thee!
For this new morning with its light;
   For rest and shelter of the night;
For health and food, for love and friends;
   For every thing His goodness sends,
Father in heaven we thank Thee!
   – Ralph Waldo Emerson

Earth laughs in flowers. – Ralph Waldo Emerson

---

*A strong body and a bright, happy or serene countenance can
only result from the fine admittance of thoughts of joy and
goodwill and serenity into the mind.* – James Allen

Where there is no vision, the people perish. – Proverbs 29:18

---

*Fasting is an effective and safe method of detoxifying the body –
a technique that wise men have used for centuries to heal the sick.
Fast regularly and help the body heal itself and stay well!*
   – James Balch, M.D., Prescription for Nutritional Healing
"Bragg Books were my conversion to the healthy way."

---

*It never hurts to brush up on the three Rs:
Respect for yourself. Respect towards others.
Responsible living today, tomorrow and always!*

If you love Nature, you will find Beauty everywhere. – Vincent Van Gogh

---

*A book is a garden, an orchard, a storehouse, a party, a mentor,
a teacher, a guidepost, a counsellor.* – Henry Ward Beecher

My father and I have shared The Bragg Healthy Lifestyle Blueprint with millions of people around the world at the Bragg Health and Fitness Crusades. I would now like to share it with you as part of the Apple Cider Vinegar Health System.

With Blessings of Health, Peace, Joy and Love,

The Bragg Healthy Lifestyle

The Bragg Blueprint for Physical, Mental and Spiritual Improvement – Healthy, Vital Living to 120

– Genesis 6:3

by

Patricia Bragg, N.D., Ph.D.
Life Extension Nutritionist

Just think, in only 90 days you can build a new bloodstream! Not a thick, sluggish, toxin-saturated bloodstream, but a rich, red bloodstream, healthy in all the vitamins, minerals and vital nutrients necessary for radiant and long lasting health. First and foremost, we must build the health content of our bloodstream. This is one of the great secrets of life: The more healthy nutrients in your bloodstream, the more oxygen is going to flood into your body, purifying its cells. Oxygen is the greatest natural stimulant. It stimulates, but doesn't depress. Unnatural stimulants stimulate, but there is an aftermath of depression. Tobacco, alcohol, coffee, tea, refined white sugar and flour and drugs (prescribed, street and over counter) have this bad effect on the body, but not God's oxygen – it's the invisible staff of life!

So, in The Bragg Healthy Lifestyle we forever discard these harmful, destructive stimulants. You are going to be strong and never allow these to enter your body again! You are going to rely on the wonderful, natural stimulants to create a more healthy vital force.

Man's days shall be to 120 years. – Genesis 6:3

First, you are going to start breathing deeper and slower, as it's important for super energy. Then you are going to eat organic, live foods, such as fresh fruits and vegetables and freshly squeezed juices, that will build up your blood health and energy.

Before you eat or drink anything, I want you to ask yourself this important question, "Is this going to build a healthy bloodstream or destroy it?" Be on the alert to protect your precious river of life - your bloodstream! When it demands liquids, give it the best – pure distilled water or live-food juices, such as fresh organic fruit and vegetable juices. Get yourself a juicer. Every day fortify your blood with fresh orange, grapefruit or carrot and green juices or combine juices such as celery, tomato, beet and parsley or see page 65. Three of the best juices to add to vegetable juices are raw spinach, cabbage and watercress. For a taste delight, add juice of 1–2 garlic buds (wrap in veg leaf to juice), excellent purifier and heart protector.

see page 65

Do not consume too much of these powerful, live-food juices. One to two pints a day is more than enough! Some people get a juicer and overdo it. Overloading your body with juices can upset your delicate blood-sugar balance. Eating the whole fruit is still the best! Just because something is good for you doesn't mean that a lot of it is. As with all things in life, moderation of your food intake is best for building Vitality Supreme!

Imagine: In just a short 11 months you will have an absolutely New You! The billions of soft cells that make up eyes, nose, skin, hands and feet, as well as all the vital organs of your body, will be renewed. You do not need to submit to the huge risk of heart, kidney or any other dangerous transplant operations!

You have within your power, through the food you eat, the liquid you drink and the air you breathe, the ability to build a fresh, vital body from the top of your head to the tip of your toes. What you eat and drink today will be walking and talking tomorrow! How wonderful our Creator has been to us, to give us the power every 90 days to build a new bloodstream and every 11 months, an entirely new body.

It's Never Too Late to Seek and Build Radiant Health!

The Creator gave us the intelligence and reasoning power to take control of our body! But the flesh is dumb! You can stuff anything in your stomach and almost get away with it until the day of reckoning!

Most young people live this way, because they believe they are totally indestructible! But what a sad lesson they learn after 40 or 50 years of wrong living! The infirmities and the aches and pains creep into their bodies, making life miserable and proving to them that their dream of indestructibility was a myth and a lie!

Live by the reasoning mind, rather than by the senses of the body. The dumb senses are constantly enticing you to do the very things that destroy your wonderful body. Look around you at the sad, broken-down human sights you see. Weak people, mentally depressed people and sickness everywhere! The average person's suffering – it's sad but true – is self-inflicted . . . a slow, self-murder!

Whatsoever a man soweth, he shall also reap. – Galatians 6:7

We should know and observe the fact that everything in the universe is always governed by definite laws. If we understand and follow these universal laws we will sow the seeds of constructive, healthy living!

Make every day a healthy day and each day you will improve! You will feel new strength and energy flooding into your body. The feelings you will experience when you live 100% The Bragg Healthy Lifestyle are indescribable! What an incredibly powerful and joyful feeling it is to be fully alive and vigorous, with unlimited energy and powerful nerve force. An amazing example is ageless Jack LaLanne who is filled with energy! (pg 35)

Weak people find weak excuses to continue living their unhealthy lifestyle. They will tell you they are too old to begin The Bragg Healthy Lifestyle Program. Age has no force, nor is it toxic! Time is just a measure. Long ago, the Bragg family gave up living by calendar years. We only live by biological years and we feel ageless.

Millions Suffer from Premature Ageing

There are millions in their 30s and 40s who are, sad to say, prematurely old biologically. Yet there are many people in their 70s, 80s and 90s who are biologically youthful, active, healthy and happy! *The second half is best.*

In our opinion, if you are experiencing premature ageing, you are suffering from a highly toxic condition and you are suffering from unnecessary nutritional deficiencies. These are the main causes of most human troubles. The Bragg Healthy Lifestyle will show you how to banish these vicious enemies. From this minute on, stop living by calendar years! Just forget your birthdays, as I do. All of us are reborn every second of the day as new body cells are being constantly created.

Cease this talk of getting old! From this minute on, you will have no age except your biological age and this you are going to control. Every day say to yourself . . .

I Will Stay Youthful, Active, Happy and Healthy!

Say it repeatedly, burn it deeply into your mind and it will sparkle all your days for your whole life!

Most people have a dreadful fear of getting old. They picture themselves half blind, hearing impaired, with teeth gone, energy and vitality spent or senile. They see themselves as a burden to their family and friends. They envision themselves in the nursing home alone, forgotten, with Alzheimer's disease.

Despite the fear of old age and the train of ailments that go with it, you can prevent this human tragedy. You can skip this terrible period by changing how you live from this day forward. Today is the day to prepare against becoming senile and decrepit. That is why I urge you to follow the wise and wonderful laws of Mother Nature. You will grow younger as you live longer! That is what this health program is all about: The preservation of your precious vital health!

Every man is the builder of a temple called his body . . . We are all sculptors and painters and our material is our own flesh and blood and bones. Any nobleness begins at once to refine a man's features, any meanness or sensuality to imbrute them. – Henry David Thoreau

Wise Prevention Helps Keep You Healthy, Youthful and Vigorous!

Lengthening life by special treatment of chronic miseries often means merely adding years of ill health and misery to a person's life. This is often called *the living death*. Who wants to extend life just to suffer? We say, the healer's function is to prevent sickness and disease.

No person is able to heal you! Only you can heal yourself! In order to be healthy it's essential to learn how to live healthy in order to be healthy always. They say –

An ounce of prevention is worth a ton of cure!

My father and I always stress to our readers that prevention is always the healthiest, best and is priceless!

Diet for health and youthfulness – Your diet should be composed of 60% to 70% raw fruit and raw or steamed, baked or wokked vegetables. By this habit, such conditions as stomach upsets, miseries and constipation, which occur often in children and adults, can be avoided (pages 32-33). Output should equal intake. You should have a bowel movement soon upon arising and after each meal.

The greatest enemy of health is constipation, but this can be eliminated by a diet that gives you sufficient bulk, moisture, lubrication and vigorous exercise of the entire abdominal cavity. In the remote parts of the world, where we have traveled beyond the influences of so-called modern civilization, mankind indulges in the normal habit of defecation after every meal. I want you to train yourself to have a bowel movement soon after arising and after each meal. Children can be taught this important habit from infancy. Living The Bragg Healthy Lifestyle faithfully, constipation vanishes!

Why not look for the best – the best in others, the best in ourselves, the best in all life situations? He who looks for the best knows the worst is there but refuses to be discouraged by it. Though temporarily defeated, dismayed, he smiles and tries again. If you look for the best, life will become pleasant for you and everyone around you.
– Rev. Paul S. Osumi, Honolulu, Hawaii

The natural healing force within us is the greatest force in getting well.
– Hippocrates, Father of Medicine

Constipation Creates Toxins in the Body

Studies reveal the presence of toxic poisons in cases of constipation. When these toxins are absorbed into the general circulation, the liver "your detoxifying organ" is unable to cope with them. These toxins are then thrown back into the body to cause trouble and sickness. Constipation and toxemia are our real enemies!

I believe that diet plays a vital role in the maintenance of health, good elimination and the prevention of disease. Research shows that diets composed of refined white flour and sugar; preserved meats, such as hot dogs and luncheon meats; white rice; coffee, tea, cola drinks and alcohol; margarine; overcooked vegetables; high fat, sugared, salted, and processed foods create many serious health problems, especially in the intestinal tract, heart and respiratory areas. It's wise to never eat refined, processed, embalmed and dead, unhealthy foods!

Your Energy is Your Body's Spark Plug

Your energy comes from the spark of life, which is maintained by the atomic energy contained within every single cell of the human body. It embodies electrons, protons and neutrons. They are constantly discharging their ionic compounds as energy is expended in work or play, whether mental or physical, in accordance with natural laws. This energy loss must be replaced. Every cell in your body is like a battery that, when run down, must be recharged. Primarily, this is done through the intake of food. Proper breathing and exercise also helps recharge your billions of cells.

Now, there are two kinds of food: The first is in a low rate of physical vibration, like the fast junk foods we mentioned: the processed, chemicalized, dead foods, as in refined white flour and sugars, etc. It's impossible to have a youthful, dynamic body when, year after year, you feed it food and drinks with a low rate of vibration.

In nature there are neither rewards or punishments – there are consequences!

Pray for wisdom in your daily living, for more faith and for more patience with yourself and others before you pray for just things.

The Bragg Healthy Lifestyle Program consists only of the **second kind of foods**: those in a **high rate of vibration**. Many have the preconceived idea that protein is the food that is in the highest rate of vibration. While protein (vegetarian protein is healthier) is an important nutrient to the human body, organic fresh fruit and vegetables have high vibrations. Fruit produces blood sugar, which helps to feed the nerves of the body. Fruit has a twofold purpose in the body. First, it's rich in blood sugar; second, it's an important detoxifier and destroyer of harmful toxins and wastes that can do the body harm.

Allergies Are Often The Body Cleansing

Often you will hear people say, "I am allergic to apples, grapefruit, peaches, strawberries, etc." These people have no idea what these foods are doing in their bodies. To give you an example, when my father was reared in the South, his typical diet was rich in animal proteins and fats from the hogs, chickens, cows and sheep they raised. At each meal, they had a wide variety of these meat proteins. I'm sad to say that accompanying these dishes were white flour biscuits and bread, mashed and fried potatoes and inevitably, a heavy, sugary dessert.

When he attended this military school (page 14) from the age of 12 on, his body became so saturated with toxic poisons, mucus and putrid food residues that, when he ate any fresh fruits, he suffered not only hives, but also colds, headaches and pains as well. These were erroneously thought to be allergic reactions. But they were the natural self-cleansing responses of his body that wanted him healthy and clean! The cleansing fruits were trying to push out the mucus and toxins through his skin, lungs, etc.!

He avoided eating these vital foods until he became a health advocate at the age of sixteen. Only after he had been cleansed and purified with healthy foods, apple cider vinegar and fasting one day a week, along with occasional longer fasts, could he eat fresh fruits and vegetables without a negative reaction.

We can change if we set our will to change. – Robert Benson

Perfect health is above gold; a sound body before riches. – Solomon

Through fasting and careful nutrition, he slowly detoxified himself and could eat all the wonderful, natural foods without experiencing the allergic cleansing reactions of his youth. His early TB was the outcome of these wrong foods. For this reason, people who have been living on a diet high in animal proteins, fats, salt, starches and refined sugars can't immediately include a large amount of fresh fruits and vegetables in their diet. It's best to slowly ease into The Bragg Healthy Lifestyle to allow the body to cleanse itself gently.

Health Transition Diet - Everyone who wants to live the healthy life must thoroughly understand just what is going on in their body chemistry. Fresh, organic, raw fruits and vegetables help flush the toxins out. The body can't be rushed. It takes the average person a long time to saturate the body with toxic poisons. Now it's going to take time to flush this debris out with this transition diet!

The more organic raw fruits and raw vegetables that you condition yourself to handle, the more cleansed your body will become! So, recognize these foods, which are in the highest rate of healthy vibration. But please, also respect their cleansing and detoxifying action!

> **We often eat 100% raw meals of fruits, vegetables or salads for a few days, but usually our meals are 60% to 70% raw:**

Breakfast: Fresh, raw juice (orange, grapefruit, or carrot, celery, garlic, spinach, etc.) or raw fruit (in season, melon, apricot, berry, peach, nectarine, etc.) or the nutritious, delicious Bragg Pep Drink – recipe page 96.

Lunch: Large variety salad with fresh greens, vegetables, sprouts and a few raw nuts or seeds (sunflower, sesame, pumpkin, almonds, pecans, walnuts, etc.) See page 97.

Dinner: Variety salad, followed by two steamed, baked or wokked fresh vegetables and one of the following: beans, lentils, brown rice, whole grain pasta, tofu (soybean curd), baked or steamed potatoes.

Remember to get your daily ACV into your diet with the ACV Cocktail and sprinkle ACV over steamed greens, cauliflower, squash, broccoli, cabbage, stringbeans, etc. It is also especially delicious on garden variety salads.

People are told they must start the day with a big breakfast, to give them great energy in the morning hours. So, they gorge themselves on processed cereal with milk and sugar; ham and eggs; or bacon and eggs; stacks of hot cakes or buttered toast and jelly. All of this is washed down with coffee, milk or cocoa. You will note that there are no fresh fruits at this meal.

Only a person doing the most strenuous physical labor could possibly burn up a meal like this, and I doubt that even they would. All the vital energy of the body will be needed to digest these heavy animal proteins and fats, refined starch and white sugar breakfasts. All too often, they lie in the stomach like a ton of bricks and have to be dynamited out. Now you know why there is so much indigestion and constipation and why laxatives are one of the biggest sellers in drugstores!

How can a big meal like this give a person strength for their morning duties? The truth is, it can't! This is how parents and, consequently, their children are brainwashed by the big food interests who sell all their commercial, sugared, unhealthy, worthless foods. You must change your ideas about food! Learn to eat in moderation. It's important you not overfuel your body. If you overfeed your body, you clog it up. A diet of healthy, organic, raw foods with a high rate of vibration will help keep your insides clean and you healthier!

51

Vegetarians are Healthier and Live Longer

Most uninformed nutritionists call meat the #1 source of protein. Those proteins coming from the vegetable kingdom are referred to as the #2 proteins. This is a sad and terrible mistake. It should be the other way around! In this day and age, almost all meat is laden with herbicides, fungicides, pesticides and other chemicals that are sprayed on or poured into the feed which these animals consume. They are also pumped full of hormones, antibiotics, growth stimulators and drugs to fatten them up and keep them from dying from the unhealthy conditions they live in!

In regions where meat is scarce, cardiovascular disease is unknown.
– Time Magazine article

Eliminating Meat is Safer and Healthier

Play it safe, become a healthy vegetarian. Look what they feed cattle – the dead, ground up carcasses of other feed lot animals who, for a variety of reasons, didn't make it to the slaughterhouse.

Speaking of the slaughterhouse scene, what kind of chemical reaction do you suppose would occur in your body if somebody put a choke chain around your neck to keep you in line, shoved you onto a conveyor belt, and made you watch in horror as all of those in line in front of you were beheaded one by one? Well, your body would be pumped so full of adrenaline from all that fear you wouldn't know what hit you! Unused adrenaline is extremely toxic. If you think for a minute that most of the meat that you consume is not packed with this toxic substance, you're sadly mistaken!

Also, consider the fact that cattle, sheep, chickens, etc., are all vegetarians. When you eat them, you are just eating polluted vegetables. Why not skip all the waste and toxins and just eat healthy, organic vegetables?

And what about that myth that you have to eat meat to get your protein? If that were true, where do you suppose farm animals, especially horses, get their protein? They are vegetarians! They get their protein from the grains and grasses that they eat. You are no different. You can get the proteins you need from the large variety of whole grains, tofu, raw nuts, seeds, beans, fruits and vegetables that God put on this planet for your health. Study the Vegetable Protein % Chart.

A truly good book teaches me better than to just read it. I must soon lay it down and commence living its wisdom. What I began by reading, I must finish by acting! – Henry David Thoreau

Whatsoever was the father of disease, an ill diet was the mother. – Herbert, 1859

Millions of Americans are committing slow suicide with their unhealthy, inactive lifestyle; heavy meat eating, high sugar and fat diets; plus smoking, drinking alcohol and doing drugs -all this damages their organs and the inside of their arteries, adding graver health problems to their lives! – Patricia Bragg

Vegetarian Protein % Chart

LEGUMES %

Soybean Sprouts	54
Soybean Curd (tofu)	43
Soy flour	35
Soybeans	35
Broad Beans	32
Lentils	29
Split Peas	28
Kidney Beans	26
Navy Beans	26
Lima Beans	26
Garbanzo Beans	23

VEGETABLES %

Spirulina (Plant Algae)	60
Spinach	49
New Zealand Spinach	47
Watercress	46
Kale	45
Broccoli	45
Brussels Sprouts	44
Turnip Greens	43
Collards	43
Cauliflower	40
Mustard Greens	39
Mushrooms	38
Chinese Cabbage	34
Parsley	34
Lettuce	34
Green Peas	30
Zucchini	28
Green Beans	26
Cucumbers	24
Dandelion Greens	24
Green Pepper	22
Artichokes	22
Cabbage	22
Celery	21
Eggplant	21
Tomatoes	18
Onions	16
Beets	15
Pumpkin	12
Potatoes	11
Yams	8
Sweet Potatoes	6

GRAINS %

Wheat Germ	31
Rye	20
Wheat, hard red	17
Wild rice	16
Buckwheat	15
Oatmeal	15
Millet	12
Barley	11
Brown Rice	8

FRUITS %

Lemons	16
Honeydew Melon	10
Cantaloupe	9
Strawberry	8
Orange	8
Blackberry	8
Cherry	8
Apricot	8
Grape	8
Watermelon	8
Tangerine	7
Papaya	6
Peach	6
Pear	5
Banana	5
Grapefruit	5
Pineapple	3
Apple	1

53

NUTS AND SEEDS %

Pumpkin Seeds	21
Sunflower Seeds	17
Walnuts, black	13
Sesame Seeds	13
Almonds	12
Cashews	12
Filberts	8

Data obtained from *Nutritive Value of American Foods in Common Units,* USDA Agriculture Handbook No. 456. Reprinted with author's permission, from *Diet for a New America* by John Robbins (Walpole, NH: Stillpoint Publishing)

If you do a complete water fast for 24 hours each week, soon you will be able to add more fresh fruit and vegetables to your diet. After a fast of 3 or more days, then you can include more foods that are in a high rate of vibration.

I faithfully fast for 24 hours every Monday and the first three days of each month. Wait until you experience this! You will greatly benefit from the inner cleansing and will love the pure, clean, healthy feeling you receive!

Fasting Cleanses, Renews and Rejuvenates

Our bodies have a natural self-cleansing and healing system for maintaining a healthy body and our "river of life" – our bloodstream. It's essential that we keep our entire bodily machinery from head to toes in perfect health and in good working order to maintain life!

Fasting is the best detoxifying method. It's also the most effective and safest way to increase elimination of waste buildups and enhance the body's miraculous self-healing and self-repairing process that keeps you healthy.

If you prepare for a fast by eating a cleansing diet for 1 to 2 days, this can greatly help the cleansing process. Fresh variety salads, fresh vegetables and fruits and their juices, as well as green drinks (alfalfa, barley, chlorophyll, chlorella, spirulina, wheatgrass, etc.) stimulate waste elimination. Fresh foods and juices can literally pick up dead matter from your body and carry it away.

Daily, even on most days during our fasts, we take 3,000 mg. of mixed vitamin C powder (C concentrate, acerola, rosehips and bioflavonoids) in liquids. This is a potent antioxidant and flushes out deadly free radicals that produce harmful effects, cancer, etc. Vitamin C also promotes collagen production for new healthy tissues and is especially important if you are detoxifying from prescription drugs or alcohol overload.

The body is self-cleansing, self-correcting and self-healing when you give it a chance with a fasting cleanse and living a healthy lifestyle! – Patricia Bragg

Fasting Removes Sludge from Your Pipes

A moderate, well planned distilled water fast (our favorite) or a diluted fresh juice (35% distilled water) fast for beginners can also cleanse your body of excess mucus, old fecal matter, trapped cellular, non-food wastes and help remove inorganic mineral deposits and sludge from your pipes and joints. (See pages 63-66 for juice fasting and combination juices, etc.)

Fasting works by self-digestion. During a fast your body intuitively will decompose and burn only substances and tissues that are damaged, diseased or unneeded, such as abscesses, tumors, excess fat deposits, excess water and congestive wastes. Even a relatively short fast (1 to 3 days) will accelerate elimination from your liver, kidneys, lungs, bloodstream and skin. Sometimes you will experience dramatic changes (cleansing and healing crises) as accumulated wastes are expelled. With your first fasts you may temporarily have headaches, fatigue, body odor, bad breath, coated tongue, mouth sores and even diarrhea as your body is cleaning house. Please be patient with your miracle body! (See *bragg.com* – Bragg Fasting Book excerpts.)

After a fast your body will begin to self-cleanse and healthfully rebalance! When you follow The Bragg Healthy Lifestyle, your weekly 24 hour fast removes toxins on a regular basis, so they don't accumulate. Your energy levels will amazingly begin to rise – physically, psychologically and mentally. Your creativity will begin to expand. You will feel like a different person – which you are – for now you are being cleansed, purified and reborn. It's truly the Miracle of Fasting – read page 58!

Fasting Brings Remarkable Results

Professor A.E. Crews of Edinburgh University, who studied both worms and animals, said: *"Given appropriate and essential conditions, including proper care of the body, Eternal Youth can be a reality in living forms! It's possible, by repeated processes of fasting, to keep an earthworm alive twenty times longer than normal and also proven with animals."* This proves the life-extending merits of fasting!

(See this important website: *www. walford.com*)

The Trail to Perfect Health

My father and I are very sincere about our fasting program. We know what it has done for us, for the members of our family, our friends, and millions of Bragg health conscious students all over the world. So The Bragg Healthy Lifestyle calls for 4 longer fasts a year, along with a faithful weekly 24 or 36 hour fast. I always fast the first 3 days of every month and all day each Monday. Also, I usually take my longer, cleansing fasts at the beginning of each season.

Remember, it took time for the body to build up toxins, so it takes time to cleanse and unload them! Take your time! Be faithful to The Bragg Healthy Lifestyle. You will reap wonderful, priceless, long-lasting health benefits. Please read our book the *Miracle of Fasting* as it gives many more details about the many benefits of fasting.

By relieving the body of the work of digesting foods, fasting allows the system to rid itself of toxins, while facilitating healing. Fasting regularly gives your organs a rest and helps reverse the ageing process for a longer and healthier life. Bragg Books were my conversion to the healthy way.
– James F. Balch, M.D. Prescription for Nutritional Healing

Eat Plenty of Cabbage – The Miracle Cleanser and Healer

Cabbage (raw) has amazing properties. It stimulates the immune system, kills bacteria and viruses, heals ulcers, and according to Dr. James Balch in Prescription for Cooking and Dietary Wellness, your chances of contracting colon cancer can be reduced by up to 60% by eating cabbage weekly. Dr. Saxon-Graham states that those who never consumed cabbage were three times more likely to develop colon cancer. A Japanese study shows that people who ate cabbage had the lowest fatality rate from any cancer. Therapeutic benefits have also been attributed to cabbage in relation to scurvy, gout, rheumatism (arthritis), eye diseases, asthma, pyorrhea, and gangrene. See our Bragg Salad Recipe (page 231). Cooking destroys the cabbages healing properties. We love cabbage and also we make a variety of sandwiches wrapped in cabbage leaves instead of bread. Try this – so delicious!!!

"Secret" of Health is Internal Cleanliness

What you want to strive for is a clean, toxicless body! Gradually include more organic, fresh fruit and raw vegetables in your diet. Have fresh fruit in the morning and a large raw, combination vegetable salad at noon. If you like, you may have some fresh fruit for dessert. Eat a yellow vegetable, such as a yam, sweet potato, yellow squash or carrots, and a green vegetable every day. Cook these vegetables by baking, steaming or wok (stir-fry) them. Always remember to save some raw vegetables for your cleansing garden variety salad.

With your main meal, at times you may have a more concentrated form of protein. My favorite, and the healthiest forms of protein, are vegetarian! If you insist on eating animal proteins, do so no more than 2 to 3 times a week. Your diet should include raw nuts and seeds (such as almonds, pecans, cashews, sunflower, pumpkin, sesame, etc.) and avocados. Enjoy beans, brown rice and legumes, soybeans and tofu as often as desired. By having a variety of God's natural foods you will enjoy a balanced diet and a healthier life!

You may use natural, cold or expeller pressed oils, such as olive, flax, soy, safflower or sesame. Read labels carefully before buying. I put Bragg organic, virgin, cold pressed olive oil over my baked potatoes, instead of salt-free butter. It's also perfect over brown rice, lentils, beans and vegetables. Foods are extra delicious with a spray of Bragg Liquid Aminos, the perfect all-purpose health seasoning (16 aminos acids) – now available in spray bottles at health stores nationwide. Also, try a sprinkle of kelp seasoning or my favorite, the nutritional yeast (large flakes – tastes better), rich in B Complex and B12.

The best way to eat potatoes is baked. I use a fast method of baking. Thoroughly scrub potato (either white, yam or sweet). Don't wrap or oil it. Bake in a 450° oven for 25 minutes. This converts the starch of the potato to a blood sugar. Be sure to eat the skin, too! Baked this fast way, it's crunchy and delicious. I don't believe in microwaves that destroy food cells, as irradiation

BENEFITS FROM THE JOYS OF FASTING

Fasting is easier than any diet. • Fasting is the quickest way to lose weight.
Fasting is adaptable to a busy life. • Fasting gives the body a physiological rest.
Fasting is used successfully in the treatment of many physical illnesses.
Fasting can yield weight losses of up to 10 pounds or more in the first week.
Fasting lowers & normalizes cholesterol and blood pressure levels.
Fasting is a calming experience, often relieving tension and insomnia.
Fasting improves dietary habits. • Fasting increases eating pleasure.
Fasting frequently induces feelings of euphoria, a natural *high*.
Fasting is a rejuvenator, slowing the ageing process.
Fasting is an energizer, not a debilitator. • Fasting aids the elimination process.
Fasting often results in a more vigorous sex life.
Fasting can eliminate or modify smoking, drug and drinking addictions.
Fasting is a regulator, educating the body to consume food only as needed.
Fasting saves time spent marketing, preparing and eating.
Fasting rids the body of toxins, giving it an "internal shower" & cleansing.
Fasting does not deprive the body of essential nutrients.
Fasting can be used to uncover the sources of food allergies.
Fasting is used effectively in schizophrenia treatment & other mental illnesses.
Fasting under proper supervision can be tolerated easily up to four weeks.
Fasting does not accumulate appetite; hunger "pangs" disappear in 1-2 days.
Fasting is routine for the animal kingdom.
Fasting has been a common practice since the beginning of man's existence.
Fasting is a rite in all religions; the Bible alone has 74 references to it.
Fasting under proper conditions is absolutely safe.
Fasting is not starving, it's nature's cure that God has given us. – Patricia Bragg
    – Allan Cott, M.D., *Fasting As A Way Of Life*

Spiritual Bible Reasons Why We Should Fast

3 John 2	Deut. 11:7-15,21	Luke 9:11	Matthew 9: 9-15
Gen. 6:3	Gal. 5:13-26	Mark 2:16-20	Neh. 9:1, 20-24
I Cor. 7:5	Isaiah 58	Matthew 4:1-4	Psalms 35:13
II Cor. 6	James 5:10-20	Matthew 6:6-18	Romans 16:16-20
Deut. 8:3	John 15	Matthew 7:7	Zachariah 8:1

Dear HEALTH FRIEND,

This gentle reminder explains the great benefits from *The Miracle of Fasting* that you will enjoy when starting on your weekly 24 hour, Bragg Fasting Program for Super Health! It's a precious time of body-mind-soul cleansing and renewal.

On fast days I drink 8 to 10 glasses of distilled water, (I add Bragg Vinegar to 3). If just starting you may also have herbal teas and try diluted fresh juices (add ⅓ distilled water). Every day, even some fast days, add 1 Tbsp. of psyllium husk powder to liquids twice daily. It's an extra cleanser and helps normalize weight, cholesterol and blood pressure and helps promote healthy elimination. Fasting is the oldest, most effective healing method known to man. Fasting offers great, miraculous blessings from Mother Nature and our Creator. It begins the self-cleansing of the inner-body workings so we can promote our own self-healing.

My father and I wrote the book *The Miracle of Fasting* to share with you the health miracles it can perform in your daily life. It's all so worthwhile to do and it's an important part of The Bragg Healthy Lifestyle.

With Love,

Paul Bragg's work on fasting and water is one of the great contributions to Healing Wisdom and the Natural Health Movement in the world today.
– Gabriel Cousens, M.D., Author of *Conscious Eating & Spiritual Nutrition*

also does. A fair priced, safer alternative is the convection oven. It's almost as fast as the deadly microwave and can be built in or placed on your kitchen countertop.

We never use table salt – it should have no place in your diet! Salt is an inorganic substance and only causes problems in the body! Organic sodium found naturally in "live" foods is best. Read labels and don't buy products that add salt!

Avoid Refined, Processed, Unhealthy Foods!

Eliminate refined, white flour products and white sugar products entirely. Eat no mushy, dead, refined cereals or those dry commercial cereals, for they are in a low rate of vibration, despite having been enriched with chemically produced vitamins and minerals. (Health Food Stores carry natural organic cereals, if you desire a whole grain cereal.)

Avoid these foods: Fried, salted, refined, preserved and chemicalized foods; coffee, China tea, cola and alcohol drinks; sugared, salted juices; overcooked, oversalted vegetables and salted, creamed or flour-thickened soups. Read page 86 for a complete foods-to-avoid list.

You now know the foods to avoid: Refined, unhealthy foods high in fat, salt and sugar; meat and dairy products; and chemicalized and sugared foods and beverages.

You now know the foods you can eat: Fresh fruits (organically grown is always best to buy or grow yourself); fresh juices; raw variety salads; fresh vegetables steamed, baked or wokked; vegetable proteins; beans, legumes, tofu, nuts, seeds, etc. If you really want animal and fish proteins, limit them to twice weekly. Occasionally, eat nothing but fresh fruits or fruits and raw vegetables for 1 or 2 days a week. Remember, vegetarians are the healthiest among Americans! Research proves this! See web: *ornish.com*

Use your imagination to plan enjoyable, live food meals that are in a high rate of vibration. Above all, eat simply. Avoid eating too many mixtures of food. Don't overeat. Be moderate in all things for the best of health.

Dr. Dean Ornish has been able to reverse heart disease in more than 70% of his patients who follow, among other things, a low-fat vegetarian diet.

Who is strong? He that can conquer his bad habits. – Ben Franklin

Eat only when you are really hungry, not because it is mealtime. Earn your food by activity, vigorous exercise and deep breathing. You will see how much more you really enjoy your food when you deserve and earn it!

The Miracle Powers of Fruits

Always keep in mind that the most perfect food for man is fresh, ripe fruits. Mother Nature, in her unique way, brings together in her fruits a marvelous balance. The fruits are living combinations of vital principles, in high rates of vibration, bio-magnetized, to release the living building blocks so necessary to maintain life.

Tinted by basking in the rays of the vitalizing sun, taking in draughts of magnetized air, drawing into itself vital minerals through its roots in the earth, delicious, organic fruits are God's perfect creations!

Man can get all the chemicals of an apple out of a chemist's dish, but he cannot construct an apple! Man may analyze all the minerals of a cherry, but he does not even know what makes it red. He may take apart and try to reconstruct a grape, and find that the grape supports life, but the broken down chemicals do not!

Fruits contain bioelectric principles that give electric sparks of life! Organic fruits are the most perfect foods from Mother Nature and God. Fruits will support life indefinitely to a superior degree when a body is cleansed and living in a natural environment. Ask your grocer to stock organically grown produce – it's the healthiest!

Who has not had his mouth water when seeing a luscious dish of delicious, ripe fruit before him - for instance some yellow pears with a dash of pink or a beautiful bunch of tapering grapes, green, red or blue? The sight of fruits and the taste of them, more so, bring an abundant secretion of digestive juices, for fruits are the most natural foods. I can say without reserve that fruits are designed beautifully for our digestive tracts.

The secret of longevity is eating intelligently. – Gaylord Hauser

Every man is the builder of a temple called his body. We are all sculptors and painters, and our material is our own flesh and blood and bones. Any nobleness begins at once to refine a man's features, any meanness or sensuality to imbrute them. – Henry David Thoreau

I have seen a sick person turn down all other foods for some freshly squeezed orange juice. His sick body craved the nutrients in juicy oranges. I have seen children torn with fever ask for fruit juice. Why didn't they ask for a hot dog? Mother Nature's guidance was in force.

But diets that consist solely of fruits are impractical for the average American, although they would be splendid for short periods in a tropical climate. While we have come so far from our natural state that we can't maintain an efficient lifestyle as 100% fruitarians, we still need to eat plenty of fresh fruits! One of the many reasons I love Hawaii are the luscious tropical fruits! Plan a Hawaiian vacation soon and enjoy the free Bragg Exercise Class at Waikiki Beach in Honolulu. It's going strong and thousands of Bragg followers from around the world annually visit the class. See info on page iii.

I especially recommend ripe organic bananas, which are not a fattening fruit, as commonly thought. They are 70% water and are high in potassium. Organic apples of all kinds make excellent eating, as do pears, oranges and grapes. In the fall, winter and spring, eat organically grown dates, sun-dried figs, raisins and apricots along with fresh fruits. When you eat fruits, see how light and wonderful you feel and look!

Avocado is Mother Nature's Miracle Food

The avocado tree is strong and insects don't bother it. It requires no spraying with poisonous chemicals. The avocado has a perfect balance of life-giving nutrients (potassium, folic acid, fiber, niacin, B6, protein, etc.). It has an unsaturated fat that helps lower LDL "bad" cholesterol. I eat avocados from my Santa Barbara orchard about three times weekly. I mash the avocado, add fresh minced garlic and a dash of Bragg Organic Olive Oil and Bragg Liquid Aminos. I dip slices of tomato, celery, carrot, turnip, cabbage, red onion, cucumber, bell pepper and lettuce leaves into this "guacamole" for a delicious healthy lunch.

Living under conditions of modern life, it is important to bear in mind that the preparation and refinement of food products either entirely eliminates or in part destroys the vital elements in the original material.
– United States Department of Agriculture

Gardenburger Creator Thanks Bragg Books

Paul Wenner, the *Gardenburger* Creator, says his early years as a youth with asthma were so bad he would stand at the window praying to breathe through the night and stay alive. A miracle happened when as a teenager he read the Bragg Books *Miracle of Fasting* and *Bragg Healthy Lifestyle* and his years of asthma were cured in only one month. Paul became so inspired he wanted to be a health crusader like Paul C. Bragg and daughter Patricia – and he has!

Patricia with Paul Wenner

Foods in a High Vibration Contain Life-Giving Substance

When you eat only foods that are in a high vibration, your body performs and operates by God's Universal Law and becomes a self-starting, self-governing, self-generating instrument! I want you to live by Mother Nature's and God's Laws so your body will be a fine working instrument for you at every age. If you have the desire to retain the vivacity, vitality, energy and enthusiasm of youth and the desire to turn back the clock of Father Time, when your body is bent, your eyes are dimmed and your gait is halting at an age when you should be buoyant with the spirit of youth, then I say:

"There is but one way to live and that is Mother Nature's and God's Healthy Way!"

With Your Hands You Prepare Either Health or Sickness – It's Up to You

They who provide the food for the world, decide the health of the world. A vast multitude of the human race are slaughtered by incompetent cookery. Though you may have taken lessons in music, painting or astronomy, you are not well-educated unless you have taken lessons in preparing healthy meals. You can either prepare health or sickness with your two hands. Healthy, nutritional planning and preparation produces healthy, delicious meals.

Juice Fast – Introduction to Water Fast

Fasting has been rediscovered through juice fasting — as a simple, easy means of cleansing and restoring health and vitality. To fast (abstain from food) comes from the Old English word fasten or to hold firm. It's a means to commit oneself to the task of finding inner strength through body, mind and soul cleansing. Throughout history the world's greatest philosophers and sages, including Socrates, Plato, Buddha and Gandhi, have enjoyed fasting and preached its benefits.

Juice bars are springing up everywhere and juice fasting has become "in" with the theatrical crowd in Hollywood, New York and in London. The number of Stars who believe in the power and effectiveness of juice and water fasting is growing. A partial list includes: Steven Spielberg, Barbra Streisand, Kim Basinger, Alec Baldwin, Daryl Hannah, Donna Karan, Christie Brinkley and Cloris Leachman. They say fasting helps balance their lives physically, mentally and emotionally.

Although a pure water fast is best, an introductory liquid juice fast can offer people an ideal opportunity to give their intestinal systems a restful, cleansing relief from the commercial high fat, high sugar, high salt and high protein fast foods too many Americans exist on.

Organic, raw, live fruit and vegetable juices can be purchased fresh from many Health Food Stores. You can also prepare these healthy juices yourself using a good home juicer. When juice fasting, it's then best to dilute juice with ⅓ distilled water. This list (page 65) gives you many combination ideas. With vegetable and tomato combinations try adding a dash of Bragg Liquid Aminos, herbs or, on non-fast days, even some green powder (alfalfa, barley, chlorella, spirulina, etc.) to create a delicious, nutritious powerful health drink. When using herbs in these drinks, use 1 to 2 fresh leaves or a pinch of dried herbs. A pinch of dulse (seaweed) rich in protein, iodine and iron – is delicious with vegetable juices.

Fasting is the greatest remedy – the physician within!
– Paracelsus, 15th century physician
who established the role of chemistry in medicine

64

Let me look upward
into the branches
Of the towering oak
And know that it grew
slowly and well.

Give me, amidst
the confusion
of my day
The calmness of the
everlasting hills.

Let me pause
to look at a flower
to smell a rose —
God's autograph,
to chat with a friend,
to read a few lines
from a good book.

Break the tensions
of my nerves
With the soothing music
of singing streams
and gentle rains
That live in
my memory.

Mother Nature and friendship are cozy shelters from life's rainy days.

Here are Some Powerful Juice Combinations:

1. Beet, celery, alfalfa sprouts
2. Cabbage, celery and apple
3. Cabbage, cucumber, celery, tomato, spinach and basil
4. Tomato, carrot and mint
5. Carrot, celery, watercress, garlic and wheatgrass
6. Grapefruit, orange and lemon
7. Beet, parsley, celery, carrot, mustard greens, garlic
8. Beet, celery, dulse and carrot
9. Cucumber, carrot and parsley
10. Watercress, cucumber, garlic
11. Asparagus, carrot, and mint
12. Carrot, celery, parsley, onion, cabbage and sweet basil
13. Carrot and coconut milk
14. Carrot, broccoli, lemon, cayenne
15. Carrot, cauliflower, rosemary
16. Apple, carrot, radish, ginger
17. Apple, pineapple and mint
18. Apple, papaya and grapes
19. Papaya, cranberries and apple
20. Leafy greens, broccoli, apple
21. Grape, cherry and apple
22. Watermelon (include seeds)

Bragg Introduced Juicing to America

Juicing has come a long way since Paul C. Bragg imported the first hand-operated vegetable-fruit juicer from Germany and introduced juice therapy to America. Before this, juice was pressed by hand, using cheesecloth. Bragg then introduced his new ideas – pineapple juice and tomato juice. Both were erroneously thought to be too acidic. TV's famous *Juiceman* Jay Kordish says Bragg was his early inspiration and mentor! Jay is going strong and healthy and inspiring millions to health.

65

Through our actions and deeds, rather than promises,
let us display the essence of love – perfect harmony in motion!
– Philip Glyn, Welsh Poet

Kindness should be a frame of mind in which we are alert
to every chance to do, to give, to share and to cheer.

Little deeds of kindness, little words of love,
Help to make earth happy, like the Heaven above.
– Julia A. F. Carney

Automated External Defibrillator (AED) Offers Fast Miracle –
for victims of sudden cardiac arrest. A recent report in the New England Journal of Medicine states that the survival rate for those who received their first defibrillation no later than 3 minutes after a collapse was 74%, as opposed to 49% survival rate for those defibrillated after more than 3 minutes. The FAA has decided to have medium to large passenger planes carry an AED. Med centers, big businesses, universities, schools, cruise ships etc. soon will have one in their first aid kits for emergencies. • www.nejm.org
Medtronic's LIFEPAK®500 AED, portable • (800) 442-1142 • www.medtronic.com

Liquefied and Fresh Juiced Foods

The juicer, food processor and blender are great for preparing foods for gentle or bland diets and baby foods. Fibers of fresh fruits and vegetables juiced can be tolerated on most gentle diets. Any raw or cooked fruit or vegetable can be liquefied and added to non-dairy Rice Dream, nut or soy milks or broth or soups. Live, fresh juices super charge your body's health power! You may fortify your liquid meal with barley green, alfalfa, chlorella or spirulina powder for extra nutrition.

The Bragg Healthy Lifestyle Promotes Super Health & Longevity

The Bragg Healthy Lifestyle consists of eating a diet of 60% to 70% fresh, live, organically grown foods; raw vegetables, salads, fresh fruits and juices; sprouts, raw seeds and nuts; all-natural 100% whole-grain breads, pastas, cereals and nutritious beans and legumes. These are the no cholesterol, no fat, no salt, "live foods" which combine to make up the body fuel that creates healthy, lively people that want to exercise and be fit. This healthy diet also creates energy. This is the reason people become revitalized and reborn into a fresh new life filled with joy, health, vitality, youthfulness and longevity! There are millions of healthy Bragg followers around the world proving that this lifestyle works!

Pure Water Is Important for Health

To the days of the aged it addeth length;
To the might of the strong it addeth strength;
It freshens the heart, it brings the sight;
'Tis like drinking a goblet of morning light.

The body is 70% water and pure, steam-distilled (chemical-free) water is important for total health. You should drink 7-9 glasses of water a day. Read our revealing book, Water – The Shocking Truth for more needed information on the importance of pure water.

Drinking 8 glasses daily of pure distilled water
cleanses and recharges the human batteries! – Paul C. Bragg

Play it Safe – Drink Pure Distilled Water!

Pure distilled water is vitally important in following The Bragg Healthy Heart Lifestyle. Water is the key to all body functions including: digestion, assimilation, elimination and circulation, and to bones and joints, muscles, nerves, glands and senses. The right kind of water is one of your best natural protections against all kinds of diseases and infections. It's a vital factor in all the body fluids, tissues, cells, lymph, blood and all glandular secretions. Water holds all nutritive factors in solution, as well as toxins and body wastes, and acts as the main transportation medium throughout the body, for both nutrition and cleansing purposes.

Since your body is about 70% water, the blood and lymphatic system is over 90% water, it's essential for your health that you drink only pure water that's not saturated with contaminants, inorganic minerals and toxins. This water will transport vital nutrients to cells and waste from cells more efficiently. This allows the body to function correctly and stay healthier!

ORGANIC MINERALS Your minerals must come from an organic source, from something living or that has lived. Humans do not have the same chemistry as plants. Only the living plant has the ability to extract inorganic minerals from the earth and convert them to organic minerals for your body to absorb and utilize.

INORGANIC MINERALS Inorganic minerals and toxic chemicals in water can create these problems:

- *Causes arthritis, bone spurs and painful calcified formations in the joints.*
- *Harden the liver.*
- *Cause kidney and gallstones.*
- *Clogs and hardens the veins, capillaries and arteries.*
- *Inorganic minerals and the toxic chemicals in water clog the arteries and small capillaries that are needed to feed and nourish your brain with oxygenated blood; the result is loss of memory and gradual senility and strokes.*

Cocktail of Toxic Chemicals

Chlorine, fluoride, calcium carbonate, cadmium, aluminum, trihalomethanes, chloroform, arsenic, copper, lead and unpleasant taste.

Tap-Water Average Contents

Water is the key to all body functions including: digestion, circulation, bones and joints, assimilation, elimination, muscles, nerves, glands and the senses.

Skin Absorbs Water, Toxins and All!

*Compared with its vast absorption through the respiratory system, skin absorption could be the major route of penetration into the body. Skin penetration rates have been found to be remarkably high, and the outer layer of skin is a less effective barrier to penetration than traditionally assumed. Factors affecting absorption are:

Hydration: The more hydrated the skin, the greater the absorption. If the skin is hydrated by perspiration or immersion in water or if the contaminant compounds are in solution, penetration is enhanced.

Temperature: Increased skin or water temperature will enhance skin absorption capacity proportionately. During swimming and bathing, it may be expected that greater hydration of skin surfaces will take place.

Skin Condition: Any insult (i.e. sunburn) or injury (i.e. cuts, wounds, abrasions) to the skin will lower its ability to act as a barrier against foreign substances. A history of skin disease such as psoriasis or eczema acts to lower the natural barrier of the outer skin layer, as do rashes, dermatitis, or any chronic skin condition.

Regional Variability: Skin absorption rates vary with the different regions of the body. Underestimated is the case of whole body immersion during swimming or bathing. The epidermis of the hand represents a relatively greater barrier to penetration than many other parts of the body, including the scalp, forehead, abdomen, area in and around the ears, underarms and genital area. Penetration through the genital area is estimated to be 100% but only 8.6% for the forearm.

Other Routes of Entry: Other routes of absorption include oral, nasal, cheeks and mouth cavity, and eye and ear areas. These routes have been underestimated in their ability to absorb contaminants during immersion in water. Inhalation serves as yet another route. In the case of swimming or bathing, the volatilized chemicals are likely to gather near the surface of the water and are readily inhalable. In addition, some may be swallowed.

* From *the American Journal of Public Health*

You Get More Toxic Exposure from Taking a Chlorinated Water Shower Than From Drinking the Same Water!

Two of the very highly toxic and voilatile chemicals, trichloroethylene and chloroform, have been proven as toxic contaminants found in most all municipal drinking water supplies. The National Academy of Sciences recently has estimated that hundreds of people die in the United States each year from the cancers caused largely by ingesting water pollutants from inhalation as air pollutants in the home. Inhalation exposure to water pollutants is largely ignored. Recent shocking data indicates that hot showers can liberate about 50% of the chloroform and 80% of the trichloroethylene into the air.

Tests show your body can absorb more toxic chlorine from a 10-minute shower than drinking 8 glasses of the same water. How can that be? A warm shower opens up your pores, causing your skin to act like a sponge. As a result, you not only inhale chlorine vapors, you absorb them through your skin, directly into your bloodstream – at a rate that's up to 6 times higher than drinking it.

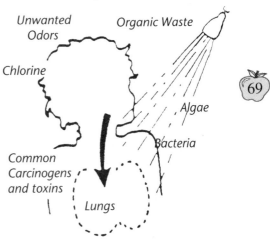

In terms of cumulative damage to your health, showering in chlorinated water is one of the most dangerous risks you take daily. Short-term risks include: eyes, sinus, throat, skin and lung irritation. Long-term risks include: excessive free radical formation (that ages you!) higher vulnerability to genetic mutation and cancer development; and difficulty metabolizing cholesterol, causing hardened arteries. – Science News

The treatment of diseases should go to the root cause, and most often it is found in severe dehydration from lack of sufficient pure, distilled water, plus an unhealthy lifestyle! See web for important info: www.watercure.com.

Five Hidden Toxic Dangers in Your Shower:

● **Chlorine:** Added to all municipal water supplies, this disinfectant hardens arteries, destroys proteins in the body, irritates skin and sinus conditions and aggravates any asthma, allergies and respiratory problems.

● **Chloroform:** This powerful by-product of chlorination causes excessive free radical formation (a cause of accelerated ageing!), normal cells to mutate and cholesterol to form. It's a known carcinogen!

● **DCA (Dichloroacedic acid):** This chlorine by-product alters cholesterol metabolism and has been shown to cause liver cancer in lab animals.

● **MX (toxic chlorinated acid):** Another by-product of chlorination, MX is known to cause genetic mutations that can lead to cancer growth and has been found in all chlorinated water for which it was tested.

● **Proven cause of bladder and rectal cancer:** Research proved that chlorinated water is the direct cause of 9% of all U.S. bladder cancers and 15% of all rectal cancers.

Showers, Toxic Chemicals & Chlorine

Skin absorption of toxic contaminants has been underestimated and ingestion may not constitute the sole or even primary route of exposure.
– Dr. Halina Brown, *American Journal of Public Health*

Taking long hot showers is a health risk, according to the latest research. Showers lead to a greater exposure to toxic chemicals contained in water supplies than does drinking the water. These toxic chemicals evaporate out of the water and are inhaled. They can also spread through the house and be inhaled by others. People receive 6 to 100 times more chemicals by breathing the air around showers and baths than they would by drinking the water. – Ian Anderson, *New Scientist*

A professor of Water Chemistry at the University of Pittsburgh claims that exposure to vaporized chemicals in the water supplies through showering, bathing, and inhalation is 100 times greater than through drinking the water. – *The Nader Report – Troubled Waters on Tap*

The power of pure water is the vital chemistry of life.

Chlorine in the water is the greatest crippler and killer of modern times. While it prevented epidemics of one disease, it was creating another. 20 years after the start of chlorinating drinking water in 1904, the present epidemic of heart trouble, cancer and senility began. – Dr. Joseph Price, author, *Coronaries/Cholesterol/Chlorine*

Don't Gamble – Use a Shower Filter

The most effective method of removing hazards from your shower is the quick and easy installation of a filter on your shower arm. We use a good filter that removes chlorine, lead, mercury, iron, arsenic, hydrogen sulfide, and many other unseen contaminants, such as bacteria, fungi, dirt and sediments. With a 12-18 month life-span, this filter is easily cleaned by backwashing every 2-3 months and is replaceable. So start enjoying safe, chlorine-free showers right away. It reduces your risk of heart disease and cancer and eases the strain from your immune system. You may even get rid of long-standing conditions, from sinus, respiratory problems to dry, itchy skin. For info on the shower filter call 800-446-1990. We use this filter and am thankful for chlorine-free showers!

Bragg's Vinegar Eye Wash for Cataracts

My 70 year-young gardener in California went to his eye doctor because his eyes were getting cloudy. He was told he needed cataract surgery! Then he began using Bragg's Vinegar Eye Wash. Now his eyes are perfectly clear and he's seeing better than ever!

Captain Diane's best friend Spike is 14½. His eyes were becoming increasingly more clouded by cataracts. Diane began using Bragg's Vinegar Eye Wash in his eyes and now they are crystal clear and Spike is a happy doggie!

Bragg's Vinegar Eye Wash:

½ tsp Bragg Apple Cider Vinegar in 4 oz. distilled water. You can use as an eyewash or as drops. Repeat 2 to 3 times daily. Keep solution in closed eyes for 2 minutes. Sometimes slight smarting occurs.

Patricia with clear-eyed Spike

Comparison of Water Treatment Methods
Steam Distilled Water is the Best

POLLUTANT	Filter Sediment	Filter Carbon	Deionization	Reverse Osmosis	Steam Distillation
Arsenic	○	○	●	●	●
Bacteria	○	○	○	◐	●
Cadmium	○	○	●	●	●
Calcium	○	○	●	●	●
Chlorides	○	○	●	●	●
Chlorine	○	●	○	●[1]	●[1]
Cryptosporidium	○	○	○	●	●
Detergents	○	◐	●	●	●
Fluorides	○	○	●	●	●
Lead	○	○	●	●	●
Magnesium	○	○	●	●	●
Nitrate	○	○	◐	◐	●
Organics	○	●	○	●[1]	●[1]
Pesticides	○	●	○	●[1]	●[1]
Phosphates	○	○	●	●	●
Radon	○	○	●	●	●
Sediment	●	◐	●	●	●
Sodium	○	○	●	●	●
Sulfates	○	◐	●	●	●
Viruses	○	○	○	○	●

○ Ineffective or No Reduction ◐ Significant Reduction ● Complete or Significant Reduction

1 – A Carbon Filter Needed (The best home distillers have also carbon filters.)

For info on reasonable water distillers & shower head filters for your home that remove harmful chemicals from your water call (800) 446-1990

The kind of water you drink can make or break you – your body is 70% water.

Exercise is Vital for Health and Longevity

Stretch, bend, lift, roll, kick and twist

To ensure youthful arteries, exercise is very essential! If you wish to live and enjoy a long, fit and healthy life it's necessary to build up your cardio-vascular endurance and start to follow an exercise program designed to keep your arteries unclogged, soft, agile and healthy. The first step is to get more oxygen into the body which will help dissolve the encrustations that have formed in the arteries. Any physical activity that injects more oxygen is going to help extend your life!

Enjoy a Tireless – Ageless – Painless Body With The Bragg Healthy Lifestyle

Don't despair in your golden years – enjoy them! My dad, Paul Bragg, said *life's second half is the best* and can be the most fruitful years. Linus Pauling, Grandma Moses and the amazing Mother Teresa, have all proven that! These three famous Bragg health followers – Conrad Hilton, J.C. Penney and foot Dr. Scholl – all lived strong, productive, active lives to almost 100 years. Countless others have lived long, healthy lives following The Bragg Healthy Lifestyle, you can too!

Conrad Hilton with Patricia

We teach you how to forget calendar years and to regain not only a youthful spirit, but much of the vigor of your youth. It's your duty to yourself to start to live The Bragg Healthy Lifestyle today – don't procrastinate! Square your shoulders and look life straight in the eye. Keep premature ageing out of your body by following The Bragg Healthy Lifestyle Blueprint. You must eat foods that have a high rate of vibration (an abundance of raw, organic fruits and vegetables) and do a water fast once a week.

It's never too late to get into shape, but it does take daily perseverance.
– Thomas K. Cureton – wellness.uwsp.edu/nfla/members/cureton.htm

Also, do some Bragg Super Power Deep Breathing exercises, get 8 hours of restful sleep at night and keep your body relaxed. Don't let anything rob you of your emotional and nervous energy and precious vital force. Do read our book *Build Powerful Nerve Force.*

Your body is being made anew every day! Premature ageing and senility result from the toxic debris that accumulates when you live an unhealthy lifestyle. Eat right, exercise for good circulation throughout your body, and there will be little or no buildup of toxins that will clog and prematurely age your body.

Cultivate and hold onto the spirit of youth *and it will be yours!* You can feel and look younger! Keep your spine straight to maintain high energy level. Daily do The Bragg Posture Exercise on page 80. Follow The Bragg Healthy Lifestyle and miracles will follow!

If you are already in the clutches of premature ageing, begin now to fight for the return of youth. Work to restore this priceless possession! You can do it! Train your body as you would that of a race horse. Follow these clear, definite instructions and you will gain strength, virility, energy, vivacity and enthusiasm! Make your life a daily enjoyment of the most precious of all earthly gifts – the power and joys of youthful, healthful living. Men and women can be young at 60, 70, 80 and even 90! Some have retained the spirit of youth beyond the century mark, like the Hunzas of Kashmir and Georgians of Russia are still doing! (Example page 9.)

The choice of which road to take is up to the individual. He alone can decide whether he wants to reach a dead end or live a healthy lifestyle for a long, healthy, happy, active life. – Paul C. Bragg

Health Suggestions for Your Daily Program

Those of you who live the incomplete life, and give up the precious qualities of human existence for dietary excesses or for the pleasures of luxury and idleness, are selling your birthright for a mess of pottage! Wake up to the possibilities within your reach! Rejuvenate your body. Make your mind keen and capable. Obey the laws of Mother Nature and God and you will see results that you now scarcely dare to dream!

Be sure that you sleep in a thoroughly ventilated, uncluttered, dust-free room, so you get a large amount of clean oxygen while sleeping. I know it's often difficult to keep dust collectors (knick-knacks, etc.) out of your home. We recently had to unclutter some areas due to dust mites. It's best to vacuum carpets often, using a hepa filter or a micro-liner bag. Put pillows and mattresses (dust mites' haven) in protective zip-closed covers. Make sure your mattress is firm and flat. Sleep spread-out to allow for good circulation. It's best not to sleep in a cramped position or sleep on your arms.

Oxygen is The Invisible Staff of Life

Oxygen is the life of the blood, and blood is the life of the body! A person weighing about 150 pounds contains about 88 pounds of oxygen. Oxygen is the most important element in the body. It is colorless, odorless and tasteless. Its main function is purification. Lack of oxygen in the body can lead to serious consequences. The majority of people are oxygen starved because they are shallow breathers. Do read *Bragg Super Power Breathing* book.

To have a healthy, youthful, vital life, we need fresh, unpolluted air in abundance, pure distilled water and plenty of fresh organic vegetables and fruits. Remember, oxygen is an unquestionable source of indispensable energy necessary for higher vital activity in the human organism! It helps ensure healthier elimination, reconstruction and regeneration within the vital factors and metabolic activities of the entire physical body.

The body is self-cleansing and self-healing! It is our duty if we want vibrant, glorious health, to do all we can to make the body work efficiently to maintain vital, super health. Not only is a healthy diet necessary, but so are good sleeping habits, outdoor physical activity, full, deep breathing and a serene, peaceful mind. We cannot live by bread alone. We must have spiritual food. And also strive for a perfect healthy balance: physical, mental, emotional and spiritual!

Through the lung functioning, oxygen is absorbed and assimilated into the bloodstream, bringing with it other unknown factors from the atmosphere. Plants, through their roots, absorb the vital elements in the soil necessary for their life. If we cut or damage their roots, they die! Man's roots are his lungs. Smokers are killing their lungs and the lungs of all those around them! Don't be around secondhand smoke – it's even more deadly! Allow no smoking in your home! See website *bragg.com* for excerpts from the Breathing Book.

We can only breathe adequately with sufficient physical movement. With the proper movements we are motivated to obtain the full elixir of life which is the breath of air. The stronger and more vigorous our movements, the more air we need and the deeper we breathe.

The oxygen in the air that we breathe dissolves and eliminates waste and builds the continuum of our cellular structure, thus maintaining our body to the highest degree possible! Each breath should detoxify and regenerate our vital forces. But this rejuvenation process must be supplemented by following The Bragg Healthy Lifestyle. Please understand that both exercise and deep breathing must be fortified with proper healthy nutrition to prevent the degenerative and destructive premature breakdown of the cells.

This explains why there is a physical decline in top athletes in their late 20s who haven't consumed a correct nutritionally, balanced diet. The average athlete reaches a peak at about 27 and then, sadly, begins to decline. I know this to be true, as my father was an active athlete for over 80 years and we saw the finest athletes reach their peak and then slowly decline, with many of them dying way too young.

Other factors affecting breathing: Our thoughts and emotions interfere with our breathing. That's why, if we have a headache or some other sudden symptom, a few minutes of deep breathing exercises in the open air will help us detoxify and reestablish our internal balance.

Actress Cloris Leachman is an ardent health follower who sparkles with health. She hates smoking, coffee, alcohol, sugar and meat. One of her solutions to health problems is to fast. "Fasting is a miracle cure. It cured my asthma."

To Rest is to Rust and Rust is Destruction!

Upon waking in the morning, stretch your legs, arms and body as you do when yawning. Continue this stretching process until you feel that every muscle has been properly and fully awakened. Good circulation and elimination are the master keys to good health! That is the reason it is important to stretch and exercise your body. Don't restrict your exercises to the morning. Make some time for them during the day to keep your circulation strong throughout your cardiovascular system during all your waking hours. Don't sit longer than one hour at a time. Do some stretching and deep breathing exercises. Get up and move around. Don't sit in a car for more than two hours. Stop the car, get out and stretch and exercise your legs and body (see page 73).

Exercises Will Help Keep You More Healthy, Youthful, Flexible and Fit

You must fight off stiffness if you want the body to feel youthful. Most prematurely old people find it impossible to straighten their spines or continually maintain good posture. Why? Because their bodies have become stiff and rigid through lack of exercise and use.

It is no wonder that men and women become prematurely old, settle down and get crusty and stiff-necked. They don't do exercises that move their spinal joints! If you have already begun to acquire this stiffness, take warning now and reverse old age habits!

Give us Lord, a bit of sun,
A bit of work and a bit of fun.
Give us, in all struggle and sputter,
Our daily whole grain bread and food.
Give us health, our keep to make
And a bit to spare for others' sake.
Give us too, a bit of song
And a tale and a book, to help us along.
Give us Lord, a chance to be
Our goodly best for ourselves and others
Until men learn to live as brothers.

An Old English Prayer

Keep Spine Flexible and Youthful

Go to work on yourself! One of the main keys to looking 10 years younger is to keep your spine active, so strive for flexibility and elasticity in every part of your body, especially your spine! Also, remember to stand, walk and sit tall because all youthful-looking people have good posture.

The spine is a marvelous instrument as well as the central support of the whole body. It is made up of a flexible column of squarish bones that are joined together with rubbery puffs called discs. This wonderful piece of equipment stores its own lubrication in little sacs at the joints. The spine was designed for action! Keep it loose and supple, and your whole body will move with grace, ease and youthfulness. Read the *Bragg Back Fitness Program* Book for the Bragg Simple Spine Exercises to help keep your spine and you flexible and youthful.

Your Waistline is Your Life-Line, Date-Line and Health-Line!

Get a tape measure and measure your waist. Write down the measurement. If you consciously pursue vigorous abdominal and postural exercises combined with correct eating and a weekly 24 hour fast (and later on, 3 to 7 day fasts), in a short time you'll see a more trim and youthful waistline. Trim waistlines can make people appear years younger. Now, let's get yours down to where it should be, if it has grown too big and fat. It's a trim, lean horse for the long race of life! I'm sure we all want longevity! Studies show the bigger the waistline – the shorter the lifespan. Living The Bragg Healthy Lifestyle is so wonderful. Life and each day is a precious gift to enjoy, treasure and guard.

People abuse their abdomens abominably! You cannot eat dead, empty-calorie foods and tell yourself that a tiny snack here and there won't show! You are completely wrong! Dead, devitalized foods create toxic poisons inside your body and this all helps to add flabby unhealthy fat and inches to your abdomen.

Nothing transforms a person faster than changing from a negative to a positive attitude. – Paul C. Bragg

Large Waistlines Lead to Shorter Lifespans

Do not overeat even healthy foods, for your body only needs enough food (fuel) to maintain health and energy. People become overweight because they have over-fueled their bodies. Studies show large waistlines produce shorter lifespans.

You are not getting away with this kind of cheating, you are just cheating (hurting) yourself! Bear in mind that as we live longer, the internal abdominal structure and stomach muscles relax more. This is called droopy tummy or visceroptosis. It's a common condition among older people who don't exercise their waist muscles. It can be a contributing cause of constipation, sluggish liver and even hernias. (Start Bragg Posture Exercise, page 80.)

When the abdominal wall becomes lazy and the consequent droop is compounded by fatty layers of flab, then trouble starts inside the abdomen. By the time most people reach 40, they have a prolapsed abdomen. Become a people watcher and you will notice that what I'm saying is true! Some need a surgical tummy-tuck (which removes excess flab) to give them a flat stomach. So, don't let your abdominal muscles droop! Make every effort to recapture firmness. It's amazing how quickly muscles respond to exercises and good posture.

Maintain Youthful Posture for Super-Health

There is a fundamental relationship between good posture and youth on the one hand and between bent posture and age on the other! To maintain the posture of youth actually means to maintain youth itself, because of the basic relationship between the healthy, normal spine and bodily vigor: the condition that signifies youth, irrespective of how many years one has lived.

The most easily recognized sign of premature ageing is the forward bending of the spine, combined with the "rounded shoulders" that accompany it. Prematurely old people often exhibit this condition to an extreme degree, almost bending over double. Even school children sometimes display early signs of premature ageing . . .

All pleasures are tasteless without health. – Fred Van Amburgh

poor posture, stooped, rounded shoulders, and sunken-in chests! On the other hand, people of advanced years, by simply straightening their spines and walking erect, appear 10 to 30 years younger than they really are. Look around you – start noticing postures of all ages and you will see what I mean!

One's entire life must be a constant fight to maintain the correct, erect position, for this gives your heart and internal organs room to operate more efficiently. Remember, the spine is the fundamental structure of the body. Along with the brain, the spine constitutes the center of the nervous system. All other parts of the body are, so to speak, appendages of the spine. Keep that spinal column straight, keep it flexible and youthful! Good health and longevity depend on a healthy, erect body. Never cross your legs – sit tall with both feet on floor. Stretch up your spine to sit, stand and walk tall. Check your body and posture (best in bathing suir or nude) in the mirror. See where you are on the posture chart – perfect, fair or poor? Start improving from today on!

Bragg Posture Exercise Gives Youthfulness

Before a mirror, stand up, feet 8" apart, stretch up spine. Tighten buttocks and suck in stomach muscles, lift up rib cage, put chest out, shoulders back, and chin up slightly. Line body up straight (nose plumbline straight to belly button), drop hands to sides and swing arms to normalize your posture. Do this posture exercise daily and miraculous changes will happen! You are retraining and strengthening your muscles to stand straight for health and youthfulness. Remember when you slump, you also cramp your precious machinery. This posture exercise will retrain your frame to sit, stand and walk tall for supreme health and longevity!

Where there is love, there is life. – Gandhi

Physical activity need not be strenuous to achieve health benefits.
– U.S. Surgeon General's Report

A strong body makes the mind strong. – Thomas Jefferson, 3rd U.S. President

I like the laughter that opens the lips and the heart, that shows at the same time the pearls and the soul. – Victor Hugo

WHERE DO YOU STAND?

POSTURE CHART

	PERFECT	FAIR	POOR
HEAD			
SHOULDERS			
SPINE			
HIPS			
ANKLES			
NECK			
UPPER BACK			
TRUNK			
ABDOMEN			
LOWER BACK			

81

Your posture carries you through life from your head to your feet. This is your human vehicle and you are truly a miracle! Cherish, respect and always protect it by living The Bragg Healthy Lifestyle. – Patricia Bragg

Remember – Your posture can make or break your health!

Stop Dying – Start Living

The Bible tells us that . . .

The kingdom of Heaven is within us.

I thoroughly believe this statement! We can make this body we live in either a kingdom of heaven on earth or we can make it a torture chamber. It's all up to you!

After childhood, the kind of body you live in is strictly up to you! I cannot live your life for you! Nor can anyone else! You are a mature adult, and you must face the realities of life. I am sure you have the willpower and desire to follow The Bragg Healthy Lifestyle, so start on the road to Higher Health today!

This is the Bragg Master Blueprint to greater physical perfection because it works with the Laws of God and Mother Nature, and they make no compromises! You either follow them or they break you! You cannot break a natural law or a God law, for it only breaks you sooner or later in your foolish attempt!

Natural Health Laws for Physical Perfection
These Natural Laws God and Mother Nature put in motion are wise, perfect laws created for your own good:

- *You must eat natural foods and never overeat.*
- *You must breathe deeply of God's pure air.*
- *You must exercise the 640 muscles of your body.*
- *You must give your body pure, safe, clean water.*
- *You must give your body gentle sunshine.*
- *You must not overwork or burden your body; this leads to stress, tensions and nerve depletion.*
- *You must keep the body clean inside and outside.*
- *You must live by divine intelligence and wisdom.*

The human body is a miracle, give it the best. Within us is the inherent potential to become perfect! It is the intent of our Creator for us to have a physically perfect, healthy, happy and peaceful long life!

Making positive lifestyle changes – daily exercise, healthy eating, eliminating stress and educating yourself about heart disease – lowers heart disease risk.
– Johns Hopkins Medical News (hopkins.med.jhu.edu/ReadingRoom/jhmn/W98/)

Enjoy Mother Nature's and God's Foods

When we are not physically perfect, we are out of harmony with the Creator's design, and therefore out of harmony with God's intent, will and law (3 John 2). In simpler words, we are, in our unhealthy living habits, opposing the will of God and Mother Earth. So, you see that to reach physical perfection, we must live correctly on all four important planes: the physical, the mental, the emotional and the spiritual. By living on the physical plane correctly, we can then reach a higher mental, emotional and spiritual state for balanced perfection.

If you eat God's and Mother Nature's foods and build a healthy, clean bloodstream, you are going to be keener mentally. The wonderful part of living by this blueprint is that we find a new calmness coming over us. You'll experience a new feeling of confidence, peace and serenity! When every cell, organ and body part is functioning perfectly, the body becomes more perfect physically, mentally, emotionally and spiritually. What complete satisfaction you will feel when you are living The Bragg Healthy Lifestyle and reaping the great rewards of a healthier, happier and more fulfilled life!

Your degree of physical perfection is the measure of your efforts in cooperating by daily partaking of proper foods, exercise, deep breathing and youthful thinking. This is your Creator's health design and intent so that you can become strong and remain physically healthy, youthful, active and of service, regardless of your age! Four exemplary long lives of service we admire: Albert Einstein, Gandhi, Albert Schweitzer, Mother Teresa.

Thousands of people every year pay thousands of dollars for state-of-the-art testing to learn their risk for heart disease. However, experts say that fresh vegetables and a health club membership may be better buys than any lab test. People who eat a diet low in fat and cholesterol and rich in plant foods, who don't smoke, who exercise regularly, and keep their weight and blood pressure in the normal range are less likely to have a heart attack than those who don't despite any predisposition or genetic tendency toward heart disease.– Harvard Health Letter

---

Spread love everywhere you go: first of all in your own house. Give love to your children, to your wife or husband, to a next door neighbor . . . Let no one ever come to you without leaving better and happier. Be the living expression of God's kindness; kindness in your face, kindness in your eyes, kindness in your smile and kindness in your warm greeting. – Mother Teresa

Food and Product Summary

Today, many of our foods are highly processed or refined, which robs them of essential nutrients, vitamins, minerals and enzymes. Many also contain harmful and dangerous chemicals. The research findings and experience of top nutritionists, physicians and dentists have led to the discovery that devitalized foods are a major cause of poor health, illness, cancer and premature death. The enormous increase in the last 70 years of degenerative diseases such as heart disease, arthritis and dental decay substantiate this belief. Scientific research has shown that most of these afflictions can be prevented and that others, once established, may be arrested or even reversed through nutritional methods.

Enjoy Super Health with Natural Foods

1. **RAW FOODS:** Use fresh fruits and raw vegetables, the organically grown are always best. Enjoy nutritious variety garden salads with sprouts and raw nuts and seeds.

2. **VEGETABLE and ANIMAL PROTEINS:**
   a. Legumes, lentils, brown rice, soybeans, tofu, beans.
   b. Nuts and seeds, raw and unsalted.
   c. Animal protein (if you must) – hormone free meats, liver, kidney, brain, heart, poultry, seafood. Please eat these proteins sparingly or it's best to enjoy the healthier vegetarian diet. You can bake, roast, wok or broil these proteins. Eat meat no more than 3 times a week.
   d. Dairy products – eggs (fertile, fresh), unprocessed hard cheese, goat's cheese and certified raw milk. We choose not to use dairy products. Try the healthier soy, nut (almond, etc.) and Rice Dream – the non-dairy milks.

3. **FRUITS and VEGETABLES:** Organically grown is always best – grown without the use of poisonous sprays and toxic chemical fertilizers whenever possible; ask your market to stock organic produce. Steam, bake, saute or wok veggies for as short a time as possible to retain the best nutritional content and flavor. Also enjoy fresh juices.

4. **100% WHOLE GRAIN CEREALS, BREADS and FLOURS:** They contain important B-complex vitamins, vitamin E, minerals and the important unsaturated fatty acids.

5. **COLD or EXPELLER-PRESSED VEGETABLE OILS:** Bragg Organic Extra Virgin Olive Oil, soy, sunflower, flax and sesame oils are excellent sources of healthy, essential, unsaturated fatty acids. (But, we use oils in moderation.)

84

You are what you eat, drink, breathe, think, say and do! – Patricia Bragg
Bob Schuller, on his famous Hour of Power *Worldwide TV Sermon,*
recently based his sermon on these words of wisdom from Patricia. You
may see and hear this powerful message on the web: www.bragg.com

The Body Must Obey Your Strong, Wise Mind

Flesh is dumb! You can put anything in your stomach from coffee to hot dogs. It is not the stomach that rules the body, but your intelligent and reasoning mind! Let me close The Bragg Healthy Lifestyle Blueprint with the unequivocal statement that the properly-directed mind can inspire the body to follow this Blueprint, thereby helping the body to become closer to physical perfection.

Morning Resolve To Start Your Day

I will this day live a simple, sincere and serene life; repelling promptly every thought of impurity, discontent, anxiety, discouragement and fear. I will cultivate health, cheerfulness, happiness, charity and the love of brotherhood; exercising economy in expenditure, generosity in giving, carefulness in conversation and diligence in appointed service. I pledge fidelity to every trust and a childlike faith in God. In particular, I will be faithful in those habits of prayer, study, work, nutrition, physical exercise, deep breathing and good posture. I shall fast for a 24 hour period each week, eat only healthy foods and get sufficient sleep each night. I will make every effort to improve myself physically, mentally, emotionally and spiritually every day.

Morning Prayer used by Patricia Bragg and her father, Paul C. Bragg

This is God's and Our Goal for You –
Radiant, Super Health! – 3 John 2

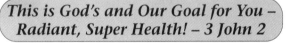

Hippocrates, Aristotle, Galen, Paracelsus, Plato, Socrates and other great philosophers, scientists and physicians for centuries have used fasting as a method of cleansing, healing and renewing the body.

Avoid all self-drugging, such as aspirin and similar drugs, pain-killers, sleeping pills, tranquilizers, antihistamines, laxatives, strong cathartics and fizzing bromides, etc. You are not qualified to prescribe drugs for yourself, and the side-effects and results can be serious. – Patricia Bragg

---

The doctor of the future will give no medicine but will interest his patients in the care of the human frame, in diet and the cause and prevention of disease. – Thomas Edison

Avoid These Processed, Refined, Harmful Foods

Once you realize the harm caused to your body by unhealthy refined, chemicalized, deficient foods, you'll want to eliminate these "killer" foods. Also avoid microwaved foods! Follow The Bragg Healthy Lifestyle to provide the basic, healthy nourishment to maintain wellness.

• Refined sugar, artificial sweeteners (aspartame) or their products such as jams, jellies, preserves, marmalades, yogurts, ice cream, sherbets, Jello, cake, candy, cookies, chewing gum, soft drinks, pies, pastries, tapioca puddings and all sugared fruit juices and fruits canned in sugar syrup. **(Health Stores have healthy, delicious replacements, so seek and buy the best and enjoy!)**

• White flour products such as white bread, wheat-white bread, enriched flours, rye bread that has white flour in it, dumplings, biscuits, buns, gravy, pasta, pancakes, waffles, soda crackers, pizza, ravioli, pies, pastries, cakes, cookies, prepared and commercial puddings and ready-mix bakery products. Also most are made with dangerous (oxy-cholesterol) powdered milk and powdered eggs. **(Health Stores have a huge variety of 100% whole grain organic products, delicious breads, crackers, pastas, pizzas, desserts, etc.)**

• Salted foods, such as corn chips, potato chips, pretzels, crackers and nuts.

• Refined white rices and pearled barley. • Fast fried foods. • Indian ghee.

• Refined, sugared (also, aspartame), dry processed cereals – cornflakes etc.

• Foods that contain olestra, palm and cottonseed oil. These additives are not fit for human consumption and should be totally avoided .

• Peanuts and peanut butter that contain hydrogenated, hardened oils and any peanut mold and all molds that can cause allergies.

• Margarine – combines heart-deadly trans-fatty acids and saturated fats.

• Saturated fats and hydrogenated oils – enemies that clog the arteries.

• Coffee, decaffeinated coffee, black caffeinated tea and all alcoholic beverages. Also all caffeinated and sugared water-juices, cola and soft drinks.

• Fresh pork, pork products. • Fried, fatty, greasy meats. • Irradiated foods.

• Smoked meats, such as ham, bacon, sausage and smoked fish.

• Luncheon meats, hot dogs, salami, bologna, corned beef, pastrami and packaged meats containing dangerous sodium nitrate or nitrite.

• Dried fruits containing sulphur dioxide – a toxic preservative.

• Don't eat chickens or turkeys that have been injected with hormones or fed with commercial poultry feed containing any drugs or toxins.

• Canned soups - read labels for sugar, starch, flour and preservatives.

• Foods containing benzoate of soda, salt, sugar, cream of tartar and any additives, drugs, preservatives; irradiated and genetically engineered foods.

• Day-old cooked vegetables, potatoes and pre-mixed, wilted lifeless salads.

• All commercial vinegars: pasteurized, filtered, distilled, white, malt and synthetic vinegars are the dead vinegars! *(We use only our Bragg Organic Raw, unfiltered Apple Cider Vinegar with the "mother" as used in olden times.)*

HEALTHY HEART HABITS FOR A LONG, VITAL LIFE

Remember, *organic live foods make live people. You are what you eat, drink, breathe, think, say and do.* So eat a low-fat, low-sugar, high-fiber diet of natural whole grains, sprouts, fresh salads, organic greens, vegetables, fruits, raw seeds and nuts, fresh juices and chemical-free, pure distilled water.

Earn your food with daily exercise, for regular exercise improves your health, stamina, go-power, flexibility and endurance, and helps open the cardiovascular system. Only 45 minutes a day can do miracles for your heart, mind, soul and body! You become revitalized with new zest for living to accomplish your life goals.

We are made of tubes. To help keep them open, clean and to maintain good elimination, add 1 to 2 Tbsps. of psyllium husk powder daily – hour after dinner – to juices, herbal teas and even the Bragg Vinegar Drink. Another way to guard against clogged tubes daily is add 2 Tbsps soy lecithin granules (fat emulsifier - melts like butter) over potatoes, veggies, soups, and to juices, etc. Also take one cayenne capsule (40,000 HU) daily with a meal. Take 50 to 100 mgs regular-released niacin (B-3) with one meal daily to help cleanse and open the cardiovascular system. Skin flushing may occur; don't worry about this as it shows it's working! After your cholesterol level reaches 180 or lower, then only take a niacin 2 to 3 times a week.

The heart needs healthy balanced nutrients, so take natural multi-vitamin-mineral food supplements & extra heart helpers – mixed vitamin E, C, CoQ10, magnesium orotate, MSM, selenium, zinc, beta carotene & amino acids L-Carnitine, L-Taurine, L-Lysine & Proline. Folic acid, CoQ10, B6 & B12 helps keep homocysteine level low. Hawthorn Berry extract brings relief for palpitations, arrhythmia, senile hearts and coronary disease. Take bromelain (from pineapple) and a multi-digestive enzyme with meals – aids digestion, assimilation and elimination.

For sleep problems try 5-HTP tryptophan (an amino acid), melatonin, calcium, magnesium, valerian caps, extracts and tea, Bragg vinegar drink, sleepytime herbal tea. For arthritis, osteoarthritis, pain/stiffness, try aloe juice or gel, glucosamine & chondroitin & MSM combo (caps & rollon), helps heal & regenerate. Also capsaicin & DMSO lotion helps.

Use amazing antioxidants – natural vitamin mixed E, C, Quercetin, grapeseed extract, CoQ10, selenium, SOD, etc. They improve the immune system and help flush out dangerous free radicals that cause havoc with the cardiovascular pipes and health. Research shows antioxidants promote longevity, slow ageing, fight toxins and help prevent cataracts, jet lag, exhaustion and disease.

Recommended Blood Chemistry Values

- Homocysteine: 6 - 8 mcm/L • Total Cholesterol, Children: 140 mg/dl or less
- Total Cholesterol: Adults, 180 mg/dl or less; 150 mg/dl optimal
- HDL Cholesterol: Men, 50 mg/dl or more; Women, 65 mg/dl or more
- HDL Cholesterol Ratio: 3.2 or less • Triglycerides: 100 mg/dl or less
- LDL Cholesterol: 100 mg/dl or less is optimal • Glucose: 80-100 mg/dl

Iron Pumping Oldsters (86 to 96) Triple Their Muscle Strength in U.S. Study

WASHINGTON – Ageing nursing home residents in Boston study "pumping iron"? Elderly weightlifters tripling and quadrupling their muscle strength? Is it possible? Most people would doubt and wonder! Government experts on ageing answered those questions with a resounding "yes" with the results of this revealing and amazing study! *www.cchs.usyd.edu.au/ESS/fiatarone/research.html*

They turned a group of frail Boston nursing home residents, aged 86 to 96, into weightlifters to demonstrate that it's never too late to reverse age-related declines in muscle strength. The group participated in a regimen of high-intensity weight-training in a study conducted by the Agriculture Department's Human Nutrition Research Center on Ageing at Tufts University in Boston. "A high-intensity weight-training program is capable of inducing dramatic increases in muscle strength in frail men and women up to 96 years of age," reported Dr. Maria A. Fiatarone, who headed the study.

Amazing Strength Results in 8 Weeks

"The favorable response to strength training in our subjects was remarkable in light of their very advanced ages and extremely sedentary habits, plus their multiple chronic diseases, functional disabilities and nutritional inadequacies. The elderly weight-lifters increased their muscle strength by anywhere from three-fold to four-fold in as little as eight weeks." Fiatarone said they probably were stronger at the end of the program than they had been in years! The results were amazing!

Fiatarone and her associates emphasized the safety of such a closely supervised weight-lifting program, even among people in frail health. The average age of the 10 participants, for instance, was 90. Six had coronary heart disease; seven had arthritis; six had bone fractures resulting from osteoporosis; four had high blood pressure; and all had been physically inactive for years. Yet, no serious medical problems resulted from the program, only good outcomes!

Exercise Keeps You Youthful, Stronger and Healthier!

Paul C. Bragg Lifts Weights Three Times a Week

A few of the participants did report minor muscle and joint aches, but 9 of the 10 completed the program. One man, aged 86, felt a pulling sensation at the site of a previous hernia incision and dropped out after 4 weeks.

The study participants, drawn from a 712 bed long-term care facility in Boston, worked out 3 times a week. They performed 3 sets of 8 repetitions with each leg on a weight-lifting machine. The weights were gradually increased from about 10 pounds initially, to about 40 pounds at the end of the eight week program.

Fiatarone said the study carries some important implications to improve the wellness and fitness of older people, who represent a growing proportion of the United States population.

Fitness Promotes Health and Longevity

Muscle strength in the average adult decreases by 30% to 50% during the course of life, mostly consequences of a sedentary unhealthy lifestyle and other controllable factors (*diet, etc.*). Muscle atrophy and weakness are not merely cosmetic problems with the frail elderly. Researchers now link muscle weakness with recurrent falls, a major cause of immobility and death in the American elderly population. This is causing millions of dollars yearly in staggering medical costs.

Previous studies have also suggested weight-training can be helpful in reversing age-related muscle weakness. But Fiatarone said physicians have been reluctant to recommend weight-lifting for the frail elderly with multiple health problems. This new government study might be changing their minds. Also, this study shows the great importance of keeping the 640 muscles as active and fit as possible to maintain general good health! Pioneer fitness crusader Dr. Kenneth Cooper of Dallas, Texas is dedicated to improving American's health, fitness and longevity. See his website: *www.cooperinst.org*

Nature's Wonder Working Phytochemicals Help Prevent Cancer

Make sure to get your daily dose of these naturally occurring, cancer fighting biological substances, that are abundant in onions, garlic, beans, legumes, soybeans, cabbage, cauliflower, broccoli, citrus fruits, etc. The winner is tomatoes, which alone contain about 10,000 different phytochemicals!

Nutrition directly affects growth, development, reproduction, well-being of an individual's physical and mental condition. Health depends upon nutrition more than on any other single factor. – Dr. Wm. H. Sebrell, Jr.

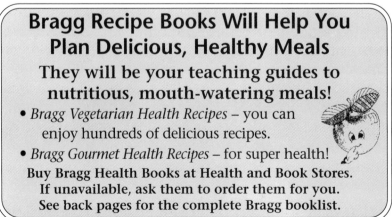

Alternative Health Therapies
And Massage Techniques

Try Them – They Work Miracles!

Explore these wonderful natural methods of healing your body. Then choose the best healing techniques for you:

ACUPUNCTURE/ACUPRESSURE Acupuncture directs and rechannels body energy by inserting hair-thin needles (use only disposable needles) at specific points on the body. It's used for pain, backaches, migraines and general health and body dysfunctions. Used in Asia for centuries, acupuncture is safe, virtually painless and has no side effects. **Acupressure** is based on the same principles and uses finger pressure and massage rather than needles. Websites offer info, check them out. Web: *acupuncture.com*

CHIROPRACTIC Chiropractic was founded in Davenport, Iowa in 1885 by Daniel David Palmer. There are now many schools in the U.S., and graduates are joining Health Practitioners in all nations of the world to share healing techniques. Chiropractic is popular, is the largest U.S. healing profession benefitting literally millions. Treatment involves soft tissue, spinal and body adjustment to free the nervous system of interferences with normal body function. Its concern is the functional integrity of the musculoskeletal system. In addition to manual methods, chiropractors use physical therapy modalities, exercise, health and nutritional guidance. Web: *chiropractic.org*

F. MATHIUS ALEXANDER TECHNIQUE These lessons help end improper use of neuromuscular system and bring body posture back into balance. Eliminates psycho-physical interferences, helps release long-held tension, and aids in re-establishing muscle tone. Web: *alexandertechnique.com*

FELDENKRAIS METHOD Dr. Moshe Feldenkrais founded this in the late 1940s. Lessons lead to improved posture and help create ease and efficiency of movement. A great stress removal method. Web: *feldenkrais.com*

If you have mastered yourself, nature will obey you. – Eliphas Levi

Alternative Health Therapies & Massage Techniques

HOMEOPATHY In the 1800's, Dr. Samuel Hahnemann developed homeopathy. Patients are treated with minute amounts of substances similar to those that cause a particular disease to trigger the body's own defenses. The homeopathic principle is *Like Cures Like.* This safe and nontoxic remedy is the #1 alternative therapy in Europe and Britain because it is inexpensive, seldom has any side effects, and brings fast results. Web: *homeopathyhome.com*

NATUROPATHY Brought to America by Dr. Benedict Lust, M.D., this treatment uses diet, herbs, homeopathy, fasting, exercise, hydrotherapy, manipulation and sunlight. (Dr. Paul C. Bragg graduated from Dr. Lust's first School of Naturopathy in the U.S. Now 6 schools) Practitioners work with your body to restore health naturally. They reject surgery and drugs except as a last resort. Web: *naturopathics.com*

OSTEOPATHY The first School of Osteopathy was founded in 1892 by Dr. Andrew Taylor Still, M.D. There are now 15 U.S. colleges. Treatment involves soft tissue, spinal and body adjustments that free the nervous system from interferences that can cause illness. Healing by adjustment also includes good nutrition, physical therapies, proper breathing and good posture. Dr. Still's premise: if the body structure is altered or abnormal, then proper body function is altered and can cause pain and illness. Web: *osteopathy.org*

92

REFLEXOLOGY OR ZONE THERAPY Founded by Eunice Ingham, author of *Stories The Feet Can Tell*, inspired by a Bragg Health Crusade when she was 17. Reflexology helps the body by removing crystalline deposits from reflex areas (nerve endings) of feet and hands through deep pressure massage. Reflexology originated in China and Egypt and Native American Indians and Kenyans practiced it for centuries. Reflexology activates the body's flow of healing and energy by dislodging deposits. Visit Eunice Ingham's website at *www.reflexology-usa.net* and *www.reflexology.org*

SKIN BRUSHING daily is wonderful for circulation, toning, cleansing and healing. Use a dry vegetable brush (never nylon) and brush lightly. Helps purify lymph so it's able to detoxify your blood and tissues. Removes old skin cells, uric acid crystals and toxic wastes that come up through skin's pores. Use loofah sponge for variety in shower or tub.

Alternative Health Therapies & Massage Techniques

REIKI A Japanese form of massage that means "Universal Life Energy." Reiki helps the body to detoxify, then re-balance and heal itself. Discovered in the ancient Sutra manuscripts by Dr. Mikso Usui in 1822. Web: *reiki.com*

ROLFING Developed by Ida Rolf in the 1930's in the U.S. Rolfing is also called structural processing and postural release, or structural dynamics. It is based on the concept that distortions (accidents, injuries, falls, etc.) and the effects of gravity on the body cause upsets in the body. Rolfing helps to achieve balance and improved body posture. Methods involve the use of stretching, deep tissue massage, and relaxation techniques to loosen old injuries and break bad movement and posture patterns, which can cause long-term health and body stress. Web: *rolf.org*

TRAGERING Founded by Dr. Milton Trager M.D., who was inspired at age 18 by Paul C. Bragg to become a doctor. It is an experimental learning method that involves gentle shaking and rocking, suggesting a greater letting go, releasing tensions and lengthening of muscles for more body health. Tragering can do miraculous healing where needed in the muscles and the entire body. Web: *trager.com*

WATER THERAPY Soothing detox shower: apply olive oil to skin, alternate hot and cold water. Massage areas while under hot, filtered spray (pages 130-132). Garden hose massage is great in summer. Hot detox tub bath (20 minutes) with cup each of Epsom salts and apple cider vinegar, pulls out toxins by creating an artificial fever cleanse. Web: *nmsnt.org*

MASSAGE & AROMATHERAPY works two ways: the essence (aroma) relaxes, as does the massage. Essential oils are extracted from flowers, leaves, roots, seeds and barks. These are usually massaged into the skin, inhaled or used in a bath for their ability to relax, soothe and heal. The oils, used for centuries to treat numerous ailments, are revitalizing and energizing for the body and mind. Example: Tiger balm, MSM, echinacea and arnica help relieve muscle aches. Avoid skin creams and lotions with mineral oil – it clogs the skin's pores. Use these natural oils for the skin: almond, apricot kernel, avocado, soy, hemp seed and olive oils and mix with aromatic essential oils: rosemary, lavender, rose, jasmine, sandalwood, lemon-balm, etc. –6 oz. oil & 6 drops of an essential oil. Web: *aromatherapy.com* or *frontierherb.com*

Alternative Health Therapies & Massage Techniques

MASSAGE – SELF Paul C. Bragg often said, "You can be your own best massage therapist, even if you have only one good hand." Near-miraculous health improvements have been achieved by victims of accidents or strokes in bringing life back to afflicted parts of their own bodies by self-massage and even vibrators. Treatments can be day or night, almost continual. Self-massage also helps achieve relaxation at day's end. Families and friends can learn and exchange massages; it's a wonderful sharing experience. Remember, babies also love and thrive with daily massages, start from birth. Family pets also love the soothing, healing touch of massages. Web: *amtamassage.org*

MASSAGE – SHIATSU Japanese form of health massage that applies pressure from the fingers, hands, elbows and even knees along the same points as acupuncture. Shiatsu has been used in Asia for centuries to relieve pain, common ills, body and muscle stress and aids lymphatic circulation. Web: *www.shiatsu.org*

MASSAGE – SPORTS An important health support system for professional and amateur athletes. Sports massage improves circulation and mobility to injured tissue, enables athletes to recover more rapidly from myofascial injury, reduces muscle soreness and chronic strain patterns. Soft tissues are freed of trigger points and adhesions, thus contributing to improvement of peak neuro-muscular functioning and athletic performance.

MASSAGE – SWEDISH One of the oldest and the most popular and widely used massage techniques. This deep body massage soothes and promotes circulation and is a great way to loosen and relax muscles before and after exercise.

Author's Comment: We have personally sampled many of these alternative therapies. It's estimated that soon America's health care costs will leap over $2 trillion. It's more important than ever to be responsible for our own health! This includes seeking holistic health practitioners who are dedicated to keeping us well by inspiring us to practice prevention! These Alternative Healing Therapies are also popular and getting results: aroma, Ayurvedic, biofeedback, color, guided imagery, herbs, music, meditation, magnets, saunas, tai chi, chi gong, Pilates, yoga, etc. Explore them and be open to improving your earthly temple for a healthy, happier, longer life. **Seek and find the best for your body, mind and soul.** – **Patricia Bragg**

Food For Thought

Fruit bears the closest relation to light. The sun pours a continuous flood of light into the fruits, and they furnish the best potion of food a human being requires for the sustenance of mind and body. – Alcott

---

The men who kept alive the flame of wisdom, learning and piety in the Middle Ages were mainly vegetarians. – Sir William Axon

---

The purest food is fruit, next vegetables, then cereals. All pure poets have abstained almost entirely from animal food. Especially a minister should eat less meat, when he has to write and give a sermon. They say the less meat, the better the sermon. – Amos Bronson Alcott

---

There is much false economy: those who are too poor to have the seasonable fruits and vegetables, will yet have pie and pickles all the year. They cannot afford oranges, yet can afford tea and coffee daily. – Health Calendar, 1910

If families could be induced to substitute the healthy organic apple, sound, ripe and luscious, in place of white sugar, white flour pies, cakes, candies and other sweets with which children are too often stuffed, doctors' bills would diminish sufficiently enough in a single year to lay up a stock of this delicious fruit for a season's use.

Through the law of cause and effect we choose our destiny through life. Moreover, we are our own prophets, for we constantly project our future state by the seeds we plant in the present. – Cheryl Canfield

DO MORE TO MAKE LIFE SUCCESSFUL

Do more than preach, practice.
Do more than think, ponder.
Do more than sympathize, empathize.
Do more than scold, set an example.
Do more than criticize, praise.
Do more than dream, make it a reality!

– Rev. Paul Osumi, Honolulu, Hawaii

HEALTHY BEVERAGES
Fresh Juices, Herb Teas & Pep Drinks

These freshly squeezed organic vegetable and fruit juices are important to The Bragg Healthy Lifestyle. It's not wise to drink beverages with your main meals, as it dilutes the digestive juices. But it's great during the day to have a glass of freshly squeezed orange, grapefruit, vegetable juice, Bragg Vinegar ACV Drink, herb tea or try hot cup Bragg Liquid Aminos Broth (½ to 1 tsp Bragg Liquid Aminos in cup of hot distilled water) – these are all ideal pick-me-up beverages.

Bragg Apple Cider Vinegar Cocktail – Mix 1-2 tsps. equally of Bragg Organic ACV and (optional) raw honey, blackstrap molasses, or 100% pure maple syrup in 6-8 oz. of distilled or purified water. Take glass upon arising, an hour before lunch and dinner (*if diabetic, use 4 stevia drops*).

Delicious Hot or Cold Cider Drink – Add 2 to 3 cinnamon sticks and 4 cloves to water and boil. Steep 20 minutes or more. Before serving add Bragg Vinegar and raw honey to taste. (Reuse cinnamon sticks & cloves.)

Bragg Favorite Juice Cocktail – This drink consists of all raw vegetables (please remember organic is best) which we prepare in our vegetable juicer: carrots, celery, beets, cabbage, tomatoes, watercress and parsley, etc. The great purifier, garlic, we enjoy but it's optional.

Bragg Favorite Healthy "Pep" Fuel Drink – After our morning stretch and exercises we often enjoy this instead of fruit. It's also delicious and powerfully nutritious as a meal anytime: lunch, dinner or take along in thermos to work, school, sports, the gym, or to the park or hiking, etc.

96

Bragg Healthy (Smoothie) "Pep" Fuel Drink

Prepare the following in blender, add 1 ice cube if desired colder:
Choice of: freshly squeezed orange juice, grapefruit or tangelo; carrot and greens juice; unsweetened pineapple juice; or 1½ cups distilled water with:

2 tsps green powder (barley, etc.)	1 to 2 bananas, ripe
½ tsp raw wheat germ (optional)	1 tsp soy protein powder
½ tsp flaxseed oil (optional)	1 tsp raw sunflower seeds
½ tsp lecithin granules	1 tsp raw honey (optional)
½ tsp rice bran	½ tsp vitamin C powder
1 Tbsp psyllium husk powder	½ tsp nutritional yeast flakes
2 dates, pitted	⅓ cup organic tofu (optional)

Optional: 8 apricots (sundried, unsulphured). Soak in jar overnight in distilled water or unsweetened pineapple juice. We soak enough for several days, keep refrigerated – also serve topped with soy yogurt. Add seasonal organic fresh fruit: peaches, strawberries, berries, apricots, etc. instead of banana. In winter, add apples, kiwi, oranges, persimmons or pears, or try sugar-free, frozen organic fruits. Serves 1 to 2.

Patricia's Delicious Health Popcorn

Use freshly popped organic popcorn (use air popper). Try Bragg Organic Olive Oil or flax seed oil or melted salt-free butter over popcorn; now add several sprays of Bragg Liquid Aminos and Bragg Apple Cider Vinegar – it's delicious! Now, sprinkle with nutritional yeast (large) flakes. For variety try pinch of Italian or French herbs, cayenne pepper, mustard powder or fresh crushed garlic to oil mixture. Serve instead of breads!

Bragg's Lentil & Brown Rice Casserole, Patties or Soup

14 oz pkg lentils, uncooked
4-6 carrots, chopped
3 celery stalks, chopped
2 onions, chopped
3 quarts distilled water

4 garlic cloves, chopped
1 ½ cups brown rice, uncooked
1 tsp Bragg Liquid Aminos
¼ tsp Italian herbs (oregano, basil, etc.)
2 tsps Bragg Organic Extra Virgin Olive Oil

Wash & drain lentils & rice. Place grains in large stainless steel pot. Add water. Bring to boil, reduce heat, simmer for 30 minutes. Then add vegetables & seasonings to grains. Cook on low heat & 5 minutes before done, add fresh or canned (salt-free) tomatoes before serving. For a delicious garnish add parsley & nutritional yeast (large) flakes. Mash for pattie burgers. For soup, add more water in cooking grains. Serves 4 to 6.

Bragg Raw Organic Vegetable Health Salad

2 stalks celery, chopped
1 bell pepper & seeds, diced
½ cucumber, chopped
2 carrots, grated
1 raw beet, grated
1 cup green cabbage, chopped

½ cup red cabbage, chopped
½ cup alfalfa or sunflower sprouts
2 spring onions & tops, chopped
1 turnip, grated
1 avocado (ripe)
3 tomatoes, medium size

For variety add raw organic zucchini, sugar peas, mushrooms, broccoli, cauliflower, (try black olives & pasta). Chop, slice or grate vegetables fine to medium for variety in size. Mix vegetables & serve on bed of lettuce, spinach, watercress or chopped cabbage. Dice avocado & tomato & serve on side as a dressing. Serve choice of fresh squeezed lemon, orange or dressing separately. Chill salad plates before serving. Always eat your salad first before serving hot dishes. Serves 3 to 5.

Bragg Health Salad Dressing

½ cup Bragg Apple Cider Vinegar
2 tsps raw honey

⅓ tsp Bragg Liquid Aminos
1 to 2 cloves garlic, minced

⅓ cup Bragg Organic Olive Oil, or blend with safflower, soy, sesame or flax
1 Tbsp fresh herbs, minced or pinch of Italian or French dry herbs

Blend ingredients in blender or jar. Refrigerate in covered jar.

FOR DELICIOUS HERBAL VINEGAR: In quart jar add ⅓ cup tightly packed, crushed fresh sweet basil, tarragon, dill, oregano, or any fresh herbs desired, combined or singly. (If dried herbs, use 1-2 tsps. herbs.) Now cover to top with Bragg Organic Apple Cider Vinegar and store two weeks in warm place, and then strain and refrigerate.

Honey – Celery Seed Vinaigrette

¼ tsp dry mustard
¼ tsp Bragg Liquid Aminos
¼ tsp paprika
3 Tbsps raw honey

1 cup Bragg Organic Apple Cider Vinegar
½ cup Bragg Organic Extra Virgin Olive Oil
½ small onion, minced
⅓ tsp celery seed

Blend ingredients in blender or jar. Refrigerate in covered jar.

Take Time for 12 Things

1. Take time to **Work** –
   it is the price of success.
2. Take time to **Think** –
   it is the source of power.
3. Take time to **Play** –
   it is the secret of youth.
4. Take time to **Read** –
   it is the foundation of knowledge.
5. Take time to **Worship** –
   it is the highway of reverence and
   washes the dust of earth from our eyes.
6. Take time to **Help and Enjoy Friends** –
   it is the source of happiness.
7. Take time to **Love** –
   it is the one sacrament of life.
8. Take time to **Dream** –
   it hitches the soul to the stars.
9. Take time to **Laugh** –
   it is the singing that helps life's loads.
10. Take time for **Beauty** –
    it is everywhere in nature.
11. Take time for **Health** –
    it is the true wealth and treasure of life.
12. Take time to **Plan** –
    it is the secret of being able to have time
    for the first 11 things.

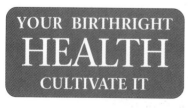

YOUR BIRTHRIGHT
HEALTH
CULTIVATE IT

Have an
Apple
Healthy Life!

Teach me Thy way O Lord, and
lead me in a simple plain path. – Psalms 27:11

The Bragg Healthy Lifestyle
For a Lifetime of Super Health

In a broad sense, "The Bragg Healthy Lifestyle for the Total Person" is a combination of physical, mental, emotional, social and spiritual components. The ability of the individual to function effectively in his environment depends on how smoothly these components function as a whole. Of all the qualities that comprise an integrated personality, a totally healthy, fit body is one of the most desirable . . . so start today for achieving your health goals!

A person may be said to be totally physically fit if he functions as a total personality with efficiency and without pain or discomfort of any kind. This is to have a Painless, Tireless, Ageless body, possessing sufficient muscular strength and endurance to maintain a healthy posture and successfully carry on the duties imposed by life and the environment, to meet emergencies satisfactorily and have enough energy for recreation and social obligations after the "work day" has ended. It is to meet the requirements of his environment through possessing the resilience to recover rapidly from fatigue, tension, stress and strain of daily living without the aid of stimulants, drugs or alcohol, and enjoy natural recharging sleep at night and awaken fit and alert in the morning for the challenges of the new fresh day ahead.

Keeping the body totally healthy and fit is not a job for the uninformed or the careless person. It requires an understanding of the body and of a healthy lifestyle and then following it for a long, happy lifetime of health! The result of "The Bragg Healthy Lifestyle" is to wake up the possibilities within you, rejuvenate your body, mind and soul to total balanced health. It's within your reach, so don't procrastinate, start today! Our hearts go out to touch your heart with nourishing, caring love for your total health and life!

Patricia Bragg and Paul C. Bragg

Dear friend, I wish above all things that thou may prosper and be in health even as the soul prospers. – 3 John 2

The doctor of the future will give no medicine but will interest his patients in the care of the human frame, in diet, and in the cause and prevention of disease.

— Thomas A. Edison

Enjoy Healthy Fiber for Super Health

- KEEP BEANS HANDY, probably the best fiber sources. Cook dried beans and freeze in portions. Use canned beans for faster meals.
- EAT BERRIES, surprisingly good sources of fiber.
- INSTEAD OF ICEBERG LETTUCE, choose deep green lettuces, romaine, bib, butter, etc., spinach or cabbage for variety salads.
- LOOK FOR "100% WHOLE WHEAT" or whole grain breads. A dark color isn't proof; check labels, compare fibers, grains, etc.
- WHOLE GRAIN CEREALS. Hot, also cold granolas with sliced fruit.
- GO FOR BROWN RICE. It's better for you and so delicious.
- EAT THE SKINS of potatoes and other organic fruits and vegetables.
- LOOK FOR HEALTH CRACKERS with at least 2 grams of fiber per ounce.
- SERVE HUMMUS, made from chickpeas, instead of sour-cream dips.
- USE WHOLE WHEAT FLOUR for baking breads, muffins, pastries, pancakes, waffles and for variety try other whole grain flours.
- ADD OAT BRAN, WHEAT BRAN AND WHEATGERM to baked goods, cookies, etc.; whole grain cereals, casseroles, loafs, etc.
- SNACK ON SUN-DRIED FRUIT, such as apricots, dates, prunes, raisins, etc., which are concentrated sources of nutrients and fiber.
- INSTEAD OF DRINKING JUICE, eat fruit: orange, apples, bananas, etc.; and vegetables: tomato, carrot, cabbage, etc.
  – UC Berkeley Wellness Letter (*www.berkeleywellness.com*)

There is a great deal of truth in the saying that man becomes what he eats. – Gandhi

Allergies, Daily Journal & Dr. Coca's Pulse Test

Almost every known food may cause some allergic reaction at times. Thus, foods used in "elimination" diets may cause allergic reactions in some individuals. Some are listed among the *Most Common Food Allergies*. Since reaction to these foods is generally low, they are widely used in making test diets. By keeping a food journal and tracking your pulse rate after meals you will soon know your "problem" foods. Allergic foods cause pulse to go up. (Take base pulse before meals and then 30 minutes after meals. If it increases 6 to 8 beats per minute – check foods for allergies.) See web *http://members.aol.com/SynergyHN/allergy22b.html*

If your body has a reaction after eating some particular food, especially if it happens each time you eat that food, you may have an allergy. Some allergic reactions are: wheezing, sneezing, stuffy nose, nasal drip or mucus, dark circles or waterbags under eyes, headaches, feeling light-headed or dizzy, fast heart beat, stomach or chest pains, diarrhea, extreme thirst, breaking out in a rash, swelling of extremities or stomach bloating, etc. (Read Dr. Arthur Coca's book, *The Pulse Test*.)

If you know what you're allergic to, you are lucky; if you don't, you had better find out as fast as possible and eliminate all irritating foods from your diet. To re-evaluate your daily life and have a health guide to your future, start a daily journal (pg 102 – 8½ x 11 notebook) of foods eaten, pulse rate before and after meals, your reactions, moods, energy levels (ups/downs), weight, elimination and sleep patterns. You will discover the foods and situations causing problems. By charting your diet you will be amazed at the effects of eating certain foods. My dad kept his journal for over 70 years.

If you are hypersensitive to certain foods, you must reject them from your diet! There are hundreds of allergies and of course it is impossible here to take up each one. Many who suffer from this unpleasant affliction have allergies to milk, wheat, or some persons are allergic to all grains. Your journal helps you discover and accurately pinpoint the foods and situations causing problems. Start your journal today!

Most Common Food Allergies

- MILK: Butter, Cheese, Cottage Cheese, Ice Cream, Milk, Yogurt, etc.
- CEREALS & GRAINS: Wheat, Corn, Buckwheat, Oats, Rye
- EGGS: Cakes, Custards, Dressings, Mayonnaise, Noodles
- FISH: Shellfish, Crabs, Lobster, Shrimp, Shadroe
- MEATS: Bacon, Chicken, Pork, Sausage, Veal, Smoked Products
- FRUITS: Citrus Fruits, Melons, Strawberries
- NUTS: Peanuts, Pecans, Walnuts, chemically dried preserved nuts
- MISCELLANEOUS: Chocolate, Black Tea, Cocoa, Coffee, MSG, Palm and Cottonseed Oils, Salt, Spices and allergic reactions often caused by toxic pesticides on salad greens, vegetables, fruits, etc.

MY DAILY HEALTH JOURNAL

Today is:____/____/____

> *I have said my morning resolve and am ready to practice*
> *The Bragg Healthy Lifestyle today and every day.*

Yesterday I went to bed at: Today I arose at: Weight:

Today I practiced the No-Heavy Breakfast or No-Breakfast Plan: ☐ yes ☐ no

• For Breakfast I drank: Time:
  For Breakfast I ate: Time:

  Supplements:

• For Lunch I ate: Time:

  Supplements:

• For Dinner I ate: Time:

  Supplements:

• List Snacks – Kind and When: Time:
                                                          Time:

• **I took part in these physical activities today:**

Grade on a scale of 1 to 10 (10 being desired optimum health)
• **I rate my day for the following categories:**

Previous Night's Sleep:	Stress/Anxiety:
Energy Level:	Elimination:
Physical Activity:	Health:
Peacefulness:	Accomplishments:
Happiness:	Self-Esteem:

• **General Comments and To Do List:**

Household Cleaning Hints with Vinegar

We don't endorse white vinegar or dead vinegars for human use – internally nor externally! But it seems well-suited for a variety of household and workshop chores. White vinegar is an effective and inexpensive household cleaner, deodorizer and disinfectant; which replaces commercial household cleaners that are full of chemicals and additives harmful to Mother Nature and you. But please remember: use only the healthiest raw, organic unfiltered apple cider vinegar (with the "mother") for all human consumption and for your skin and hair.

VINEGAR USES FOR KITCHEN CLEANING

• **Appliances and Countertops:** clean and disinfect with vinegar-dampened sponge or cloth.

• **Greasy Areas:** mix ¼ cup vinegar with 2 cups hot water and add 1 to 2 dashes of biodegradable liquid soap. (Keep mixture in handy, labeled spray bottle.)

• **Sponges and Dish Rags:** disinfect and deodorize by soaking overnight in 1 quart hot water with ¼ cup vinegar.

• **Chopping and Bread Boards:** wipe down with full-strength white vinegar to disinfect; or sprinkle with baking soda before spraying with vinegar, wait 30 minutes before wiping clean, then rinse with water.

• **Pots and Pans:** clean and polish with paste of baking soda and vinegar. Remove stubborn, stuck-on food with a 50/50 vinegar-water soak.

• **Glass and China:** stop spotting by mixing ½ cup vinegar in dishwater, or by placing 1 cup vinegar on bottom rack of electric dishwasher before starting wash.

• **Drains and Pipes:** keep fresh-smelling and free-flowing with ½ cup of baking soda followed by ½ cup of vinegar. Cover drain opening with plate for an hour or longer before flushing through with cold water.

• **Garbage Disposals:** keep clean by grinding up frozen vinegar ice cubes (80/20 vinegar-water solution to make cleansing ice cubes).

Of all the gifts that a wise providence grants us to make life fuller and happier – friendship is the most beautiful. – Epicurus

The secret of longevity largely is eating intelligently. – Gayelord Hauser

VINEGAR USES FOR THE BATHROOM

• **Chrome and Stainless Steel:** straight vinegar will disinfect and polish fixtures; apply with sponge, then buff with soft cloth.

• **Toilet Bowl:** use ½ cup straight vinegar, let stand an hour or more and flush. For bad stains, follow vinegar with sprinkle of biodegradable cleanser; after 2 hours brush and flush. If stains persist use Clorox bleach (½ cup) overnight.

• **Sink, Tub and Shower:** spray with 80/20 vinegar-water mixture, leave 5 minutes, then scrub and rinse.

• **Shower Curtains:** put through washer rinse cycle with 1 to 2 cups vinegar. Spray with 50/50 vinegar-water solution to help prevent mold.

• **Garbage Pails:** disinfect with a warm water and vinegar solution. Let set for an hour or overnight.

VINEGAR USES FOR THE LAUNDRY ROOM

• **Washer Tub and Hoses:** remove soap accumulations by running machine for full cycle with pint of vinegar.

• **New Clothes, Linens, etc:** to remove manufacturing chemicals and new smell odors, add 1 to 2 cups vinegar to first wash before using.

• **Perspiration Odor and Stained Clothes:** soak overnight in ¼ cup vinegar and enough water to cover or soak in washer or pan, then wash in morning.

• **Clothes Final Rinse Cycle:** to help remove static and lint add ½ cup vinegar.

• **To Soften and Disinfect Fabric, Clothes etc:** add ¼ cup vinegar to most loads.

• **Fruit and Grass Stains:** dab with straight vinegar within 24 hours to safely remove most stains and spots.

• **Musky Smells:** to remove odor and freshen clean cotton clothes just sprinkle with vinegar and press.

• **Steam Iron Plate:** to eliminate mineral deposits, fill iron reservoir with straight vinegar and allow to steam on rag, then fill with plain water and turn upside down and drain.

• **Scorched Fabric:** gently rub with vinegar, then wipe with clean, white cloth.

Never underestimate the power of a kind word or deed.

VINEGAR USES FOR FLOORS, WALLS & FURNITURE

• **Windows:** spray 50/50 vinegar-water mixture, then wipe clean with squeegee. (Great for eye glasses.)

• **Floors:** sponge mop with 1 cup of vinegar in a bucket of warm water. Also removes dull residue left by most commercial cleaners.

• **Carpets:** light stains are extracted using a mix of 2 Tbsps. salt and ½ cup vinegar; rub paste into carpet and allow to dry before vacuuming.

• **Furniture:** remove cloudy look & brighten by rubbing with a mixture of 1 Tbsps. vinegar in a quart of warm water, then buff with soft cloth. Remove white rings from tables with a mixture of equal parts vinegar and olive oil.

• **Vinyl Surfaces:** wipe down with 2 Tbsps. liquid soap and ½ cup vinegar before rinsing with water and drying.

• **Toys:** Clean and disinfect with a light spray of vinegar (50/50 vinegar-water solution) and brush or wipe clean.

• **Air Freshener:** mask kitchen odors by simmering a pot of water with ½ cup vinegar.

VINEGAR USES FOR OUTSIDE

• **Car & Car Windows:** keep frost-free with coating solution of 50/50 vinegar to water. Also, dissolve old decals and chewing gum with straight vinegar.

• **Paint Brushes:** soften by soaking in boiling vinegar; also, remember that vinegar absorbs paint odors!

• **Ants:** spray equal parts vinegar and water on areas where an ant invasion might or has occurred; vinegar works as a non-toxic "pesticide."

• **Fresh-Cut Flowers:** preserve by adding 2 Tbsps. vinegar to quart of warm water in flower vase.

• **Unwanted Grass & Weeds:** pour on straight vinegar.

God will not change the condition of men,
until they change what is in themselves. – Koran

There is no such thing as too many friends, just as there
is never too much happiness! – Jean de La Bruyere

Happiness is a rainbow in your heart – a real health sparkler!
– Patricia Bragg

Our Favorite Quotes We Share with You . . .
where space allows. We all need inspiring, informative words of wisdom to help guide us in our daily living.

Here's a wise ancient Turkish saying: No matter how far you've gone down on a wrong road, turn back and get on the right road!

I cannot overstate the importance of the habit of quiet meditation and prayer for more health of body, mind and spirit. – Patricia Bragg

Breathing is the movement of spirit within the body; and working with breathing is a form of spiritual practice. – Andrew Weil, M.D.

Dream big, think big, but enjoy the small miracles of everyday life.

When you live The Bragg Healthy Lifestyle *you activate your own powerful internal defense arsenal and help maintain it at top efficiency.*

We are recharged and blessed by each one of you reading our teachings. They are filled with health wisdom and love for you. – thank you! – Patricia Bragg

Earn Your Bragging Rights
Live The Bragg Healthy Lifestyle
To Attain Super Health & Enjoy Longevity

Health Crusaders Paul Bragg and daughter Patricia traveled the world spreading health, inspiring millions to renew and revitalize their health.

The Bragg books are written to inspire and guide you to health, fitness and longevity. Remember, the book you don't read won't help. So please read and reread the Bragg Books and live The Bragg Healthy Lifestyle!

With Blessings of Health, Peace, Joy and Love,

Patricia and Paul

Index

"I conceive that a knowledge of books is the basis on which all other knowledge rests." – George Washington, 1st U.S. President

Kindness should be a frame of mind in which we are alert to every opportunity: to do, to give, to share and to cheer. – Patricia Bragg

Index

Always do what is right – despite any public opinions.

What sunshine is to flowers, smiles are to humanity. – Joseph Addison

**HAVE AN
APPLE
HEALTHY LIFE!**

Who you are speaks so loudly, I can't hear what you're saying.
– Ralph Waldo Emerson

*Love is not a matter of counting the years –
it's making the years count.* – William Smith

GO ORGANIC! DON'T PANIC! — eat fruits • vegetables • BRAGG — GUARD YOUR TOTAL HEALTH

FROM THE AUTHORS

This book was written for You! It can be your passport to a healthy, long, vital life. We in the Alternative Health Therapies join hands in one common objective – promoting a high standard of health for everyone. Healthy nutrition points the way – which is Mother Nature and God's Way. This book teaches you how to work with them, not against them. Health Doctors, therapists nurses, teachers and caregivers are becoming more dedicated than ever to keeping their patients healthy and fit. This book was written to emphasize the great needed importance of living a lifetime of healthy living, close to Mother Nature and God.

Statements in this book are scientific health findings, known facts of physiology and biological therapeutics. Paul C. Bragg practiced the natural methods of living for over 80 years with highly beneficial results, knowing that they were safe and of great value. His daughter Patricia lectured and co-authored the Bragg Books with him and continues to carry on The Bragg Health Crusades.

Paul C. Bragg and daughter Patricia express their opinions solely as Public Health Educators and Health Crusaders. They offer no cure for disease. Only the body has the ability to cure a person. Experts may disagree with some of the statements made in this book. However, such statements are considered to be factual, based on the long-time health experience of pioneers Paul C. Bragg and Patricia Bragg. If you suspect you have a health problem, please seek qualified health professionals to help you make the healthiest, wisest and best-informed choices.

Oxygen is the main nutrient of the body. When we improve our oxygen intake, with exercise and full deep breathing we enhance our immune system and the body's ability to detoxify and stay healthy. – Dr. Michael Schachter, Columbia
www.mbschachter.com

Be sure you get calcium and magnesium together, because magnesium helps your body to metabolize calcium. Seeds, nuts and natural nut butters contain magnesium, of which you require about 300 mg. daily. Potassium is another heart – healthy mineral that lowers blood pressure and helps prevent strokes.

Your resting pulse (at times when you're not exercising) will slow down with regular exercise, a sign that it's becoming more efficient. An unfit person's resting pulse will probably be around 75. Your goal should be around 60.

Send for Free Health Bulletins

Patricia Bragg wants to keep in touch with you, your relatives and friends about the latest Health, Nutrition, Exercise and Longevity Discoveries. Please enclose one stamp for each USA name listed. Foreign listings send postal reply coupons.

With Blessings of Health and Thanks,

Patricia

Please make copy, then print clearly and mail to:

BRAGG HEALTH CRUSADES, Box 7, Santa Barbara, CA 93102
You can help too!
Keep the Bragg Health Crusades "Crusading" with your tax-deductible gifts.

Name _____

Address _____ Apt. No. _____

City _____ State _____ Zip _____

Phone ( ) _____ E-mail _____

Name _____

Address _____ Apt. No. _____

City _____ State _____ Zip _____

Phone ( ) _____ E-mail _____

Name _____

Address _____ Apt. No. _____

City _____ State _____ Zip _____

Phone ( ) _____ E-mail _____

Name _____

Address _____ Apt. No. _____

City _____ State _____ Zip _____

Phone ( ) _____ E-mail _____

Name _____

Address _____ Apt. No. _____

City _____ State _____ Zip _____

Phone ( ) _____ E-mail _____

Bragg Health Crusades spreading health worldwide since 1912

BRAGG "HOW-TO, SELF-HEALTH" BOOKS

Authored by America's First Family of Health
Live Longer – Healthier – Stronger Self-Improvement Library

Qty.	Bragg Book Titles	ORDER FORM	Health Science ISBN 0-87790	Price	$ Total
____	**Apple Cider Vinegar** – Miracle Health System (over 6 million in print)			6.95	.
____	**Bragg Healthy Lifestyle** – Vital Living to 120 (formerly Toxicless Diet)			7.95	.
____	**Super Power Breathing** for Super Energy and High Health			7.95	.
____	**Miracle of Fasting** – Bragg Bible of Health for longevity & physical rejuvenation ...			8.95	.
____	**Water – The Shocking Truth** (learn safest water to drink & why)			7.95	.
____	**Bragg Gourmet Health Recipes** for Super Health			9.95	.
____	**Build Powerful Nerve Force** (reduce fatigue, stress, anger, anxiety)			8.95	.
____	**Healthy Heart & Cardiovascular System** – Have a fit heart at any age			8.95	.
____	**Bragg Back Fitness Program** for pain-free strong back			7.95	.

Total Copies   Prices subject to change without notice.

TOTAL BOOKS $	.
CA Residents add sales tax	.
Shipping & Handling	.

These books will soon be in print.
Call (800) 446-1990 to check availability.

TOTAL ENCLOSED $
(USA Funds Only)   .

- **Bragg Vegetarian Recipes** – $9.95
  (new version of the old favorite) for Super Health
- **Healthy Eye/Vision Program** – $8.95
  – Improve and Protect Your Eyesight
- **Build Healthy, Strong Feet** – $8.95
  – "Best Complete Foot Progam." – Dr. Scholl

USA Shipping	Please add $4 first book $1 each additional book

USA retail book orders over $50 add $6 only

Foreign Shipping	Canada & Foreign orders add $5 first book, $1.50 @ additional book

Please Specify: ☐ Money Order ☐ Cash ☐ Check

Charge To: ☐ Visa ☐ Master Card ☐ Discover

Credit Card Number: ___ ___ ___ ___ — ___ ___ ___ ___ — ___ ___ ___ ___ — ___ ___ ___ ___   Card Expires: Month ___ Year ___

Signature: _____

CREDIT CARD ORDERS ONLY
CALL **(800) 446-1990**
OR FAX **(805) 968-1001**

Business office calls **(805) 968-1020.** We accept MasterCard Discover or VISA phone orders. Please prepare your order using this order form. It will speed your call and serve as your order record. Hours: 8 am to 4 pm Pacific Time, Monday thru Thursday.
Visit our Website: http://www.bragg.com & e-mail: books@bragg.com

See & Order Bragg 'Bound' Books, E-Books, & Products on Bragg Website.
Now Bragg E-Books are available 50% off at bragg.com.

Mail to: **HEALTH SCIENCE, Box 7, Santa Barbara, CA 93102 USA**

Name
_____

Address _____   Apt. No. _____

City _____   State _____   Zip _____

Phone (___) _____   ● E-mail _____   BOF 5-02

BRAGG ORGANIC APPLE CIDER VINEGAR

SIZE	PRICE	USA SHIPPING & HANDLING	AMT	$ TOTAL
16 oz.	$ 2.19 each	Please add $6 for 1st bottle and $1.50 each additional bottle		.
16 oz.	$21.00 Spec./12	S/H Cost by Time Zone: CA $8. PST/MST $10. CST $14. EST $16.		.
32 oz.	$ 3.79 each	Please add $6 for 1st bottle and $2.00 each additional bottle.		.
32 oz.	$40.00 Spec./12	S/H Cost by Time Zone: CA $12. PST/MST $16. CST $24. EST $28.		.

Bragg Vinegar is a food and not taxable

Vinegar	$.
Shipping & Handling	.
TOTAL $	.

BRAGG LIQUID AMINOS

SIZE	PRICE	USA SHIPPING & HANDLING	AMT	$ TOTAL
6 oz.	$2.98 each	Please add $4.00 for 1st 3 bottles – $1.25 each additional bottle.		.
6 oz.	$65.00 Spec./24	S/H Cost by Time Zone: CA $8. PST/MST $9. CST $10. EST $12.		.
16 oz.	$3.95 each	Please add $6 for 1st bottle – $1.25 each additional bottle.		.
16 oz.	$42.00 Spec./12	S/H Cost by Time Zone: CA $8. PST/MST $9. CST $12. EST $13.		.
32 oz.	$6.45 each	Please add $6 for 1st bottle – $2.00 each additional bottle.		.
32 oz.	$70.00 Spec./12	S/H Cost by Time Zone: CA $10. PST/MST $13. CST $19. EST $23.		.

Bragg Aminos is a food and not taxable

Aminos	$.
Shipping & Handling	.
TOTAL $	.

BRAGG ORGANIC OLIVE OIL

SIZE	PRICE	USA SHIPPING & HANDLING	AMT	$ TOTAL
12.7 oz.	$6.78 each	Please add $6 for 1st bottle and $1.25 each additional bottle.		.
12.7 oz.	$30.00 Spec./6	S/H Cost by Time Zone: CA $6. PST/MST $7. CST $8 EST $9.		.
12.7 oz.	$58.00 Spec./12	S/H Cost by Time Zone: CA $8. PST/MST $9. CST $12. EST $15.		.

Bragg Olive Oil is a food and not taxable

Olive Oil	$.
Shipping & Handling	.
TOTAL $	.

Foreign orders, please inquire on postage

Please Specify: ☐ Check ☐ Money Order ☐ Cash
Charge To: ☐ Visa ☐ MasterCard ☐ Discover

Credit Card
Number: _ _ _ _ — _ _ _ _ — _ _ _ _ — _ _ _ _   Card Expires: ___/___
Month / Year

MasterCard VISA DISCOVER Signature: _____

CREDIT CARD ORDERS ONLY
CALL **(800) 446-1990**
OR FAX **(805) 968-1001**

Business office calls (805) 968-1020. We accept MasterCard Discover or VISA phone orders. Please prepare your order using this order form. It will speed your call and serve as your order record. Hours: 8 am to 4 pm Pacific Time, Monday through Thursday.
Visit our Web Site: http://www.bragg.com & e-mail: orders@bragg.com

Mail to: **HEALTH SCIENCE, Box 7, Santa Barbara, CA 93102 USA**

Please Print or Type – Be sure to give street & house number to facilitate delivery.

Name _____

Address _____ Apt. No. _____

City _____ State _____ Zip _____

(___) _____
Phone   E-mail   BOF 5-02

Bragg Health Products are available at most Health Stores.

BRAGG "HOW-TO, SELF-HEALTH" BOOKS

Authored by America's First Family of Health
Live Longer – Healthier – Stronger Self-Improvement Library

Qty.	Bragg Book Titles ORDER FORM Health Science ISBN 0-87790	Price	$ Total
_____	**Apple Cider Vinegar** – Miracle Health System (over 6 million in print)	6.95	.
_____	**Bragg Healthy Lifestyle** – Vital Living to 120 (formerly Toxicless Diet).......	7.95	.
_____	**Super Power Breathing** for Super Energy and High Health	7.95	.
_____	**Miracle of Fasting** – Bragg Bible of Health for longevity & physical rejuvenation ...	8.95	.
_____	**Water – The Shocking Truth** (learn safest water to drink & why)	7.95	.
_____	**Bragg Gourmet Health Recipes** for Super Health	9.95	.
_____	**Build Powerful Nerve Force** (reduce fatigue, stress, anger, anxiety)	8.95	.
_____	**Healthy Heart & Cardiovascular System** – Have a fit heart at any age	8.95	.
	Bragg Back Fitness Program for pain-free strong back	7.95	.

Total Copies   Prices subject to change without notice.

TOTAL BOOKS $.

These books will soon be in print.
Call (800) 446-1990 to check availability.

CA Residents add sales tax .

Shipping & Handling .

- **Bragg Vegetarian Recipes – $9.95**
  (new version of the old favorite) for Super Health
- **Healthy Eye/Vision Program – $8.95**
  – Improve and Protect Your Eyesight
- **Build Healthy, Strong Feet – $8.95**
  – "Best Complete Foot Progam." – Dr. Scholl

TOTAL ENCLOSED
(USA Funds Only) $.

USA Shipping Please add $4 first book $1 each additional book

USA retail book orders over $50 add $6 only

Please Specify: ☐ Money Order   ☐ Cash   ☐ Check

Foreign Shipping Canada & Foreign orders add $5 first book, $1.50 @ additional book

Charge To: ☐ Visa   ☐ Master Card   ☐ Discover

Credit Card Number: _ _ _ _ — _ _ _ _ — _ _ _ _ — _ _ _ _   Card Expires: | (Month Year)

Signature:_____

CREDIT CARD ORDERS ONLY
CALL **(800) 446-1990**
OR FAX **(805) 968-1001**

Business office calls (805) 968-1020. We accept MasterCard Discover or VISA phone orders. Please prepare your order using this order form. It will speed your call and serve as your order record. Hours: 8 am to 4 pm Pacific Time, Monday thru Thursday.
Visit our Website: http://www.bragg.com & e-mail: books@bragg.com

See & Order Bragg 'Bound' Books, E-Books, & Products on Bragg Website.
Now Bragg E-Books are available 50% off at www.bragg.com.

Mail to: **HEALTH SCIENCE, Box 7, Santa Barbara, CA 93102 USA**

Name _____

Address _____ Apt. No. _____

City _____ State _____ Zip _____

Phone (_____) ● E-mail _____   BOF 5-02

Bragg Books are available most Health & Book Stores – Nationwide

Send for Free Health Bulletins

Patricia Bragg wants to keep in touch with you, your relatives and friends about the latest Health, Nutrition, Exercise and Longevity Discoveries. Please enclose one stamp for each USA name listed. Foreign listings send postal reply coupons.

With Blessings of Health and Thanks,

Patricia

Please make copy, then print clearly and mail to:

BRAGG HEALTH CRUSADES, Box 7, Santa Barbara, CA 93102
You can help too!
Keep the Bragg Health Crusades "Crusading" with your tax-deductible gifts.

Name

Address   Apt. No.

City   State   Zip

Phone (   )   E-mail

Name

Address   Apt. No.

City   State   Zip

Phone (   )   E-mail

Name

Address   Apt. No.

City   State   Zip

Phone (   )   E-mail

Name

Address   Apt. No.

City   State   Zip

Phone (   )   E-mail

Name

Address   Apt. No.

City   State   Zip

Phone (   )   E-mail

Bragg Health Crusades spreading health worldwide since 1912

PAUL C. BRAGG, N.D., Ph.D.
Life Extension Specialist • World Health Crusader
Lecturer and Advisor to Olympic Athletes, Royalty and Stars
Originator of Health Food Stores – Now Worldwide

For almost a Century, Living Proof that his
"Health and Fitness Way of Life" Works Wonders!

Paul C. Bragg, Father of the Health Movement in America, had vision and dedication. This dynamic Crusader for worldwide health and fitness is responsible for more *firsts* in the history of the Health Movement than any other individual.

Bragg's amazing pioneering achievements the world now enjoys:

- Bragg originated, named and opened the first Health Food Store in America.
- Bragg Health Crusades pioneered the first Health Lectures across America. Bragg inspired followers to open Health Stores across America and also worldwide.
- Bragg was the first to introduce pineapple juice and tomato juice to America.
- He introduced Juice Therapy in America by importing the first hand-juicers.
- He was the first to introduce and distribute honey and date sugar nationwide.
- Bragg pioneered Radio Health Programs from Hollywood three times daily in the 20s.
- Bragg and daughter Patricia pioneered a Health TV show from Hollywood to spread The Bragg Health Crusade on their show, *Health and Happiness*. It included exercises, health recipes, visual demonstrations and guest appearances by famous, health-minded people.
- Bragg opened the first health restaurants and the first health spas in America.
- He created the first health foods and products and then made them available nationwide: herbal teas, health beverages, seven-grain cereals and crackers, health cosmetics, health candies, calcium, vitamins and mineral supplements, wheat germ, digestive enzymes from papaya, herbs and kelp seasonings, and amino acids from soybeans. Bragg inspired others to follow (Schiff, Shaklee, Twin Labs, Herbalife, etc.) and now thousands of health items are available worldwide!

Crippled by TB as a teenager, Bragg developed his own eating, breathing and exercising program to rebuild his body into an ageless, tireless, pain-free citadel of glowing, super health. He excelled in running, swimming, biking, progressive weight training and mountain climbing. He made an early pledge to God, in return for his renewed health, to spend the rest of his life showing others the road to super health. He honored his pledge! Paul Bragg's health pioneering made a difference worldwide.

A legend and beloved health crusader to millions, Bragg was the inspiration and personal health and fitness advisor to top Olympic Stars from 4-time swimming Gold Medalist Murray Rose to 3-time track Gold Medalist Betty Cuthbert of Australia, his relative (pole-vaulting Gold Medalist), Don Bragg and countless others. Jack LaLanne, the original TV Fitness King , says, *"Bragg saved my life at age 15 when I attended the Bragg Crusade in Oakland, California."* From the earliest days, Bragg advised the greatest Hollywood Stars and giants of American Business. J. C. Penney, Del E. Webb, Dr. Scholl and Conrad Hilton are just a few who he inspired to long, successful, healthy, active lives!

Dr. Bragg changed the lives of millions worldwide in all walks of life with the Bragg Health Crusades, Books, Radio and TV appearances. (See and hear him on the web.)

BRAGG HEALTH CRUSADES, Box 7, SANTA BARBARA, CA 93102 USA • www.bragg.com

PATRICIA BRAGG, N.D., Ph.D.
Health Crusader & Angel of Health & Healing

**Author, Lecturer, Nutritionist, Health Educator & Fitness Advisor
to World Leaders, Hollywood Stars, Singers, Dancers, Athletes, etc.**

Patricia is a 100% dedicated health crusader with a passion like her father, Paul C. Bragg, world renowned health authority. Patricia has won international fame on her own in this field. She conducts Health and Fitness Seminars for Women's, Men's, Youth and Church Groups throughout the world . . . and promotes Bragg "How-To, Self-Health" Books in Lectures, on Radio and Television Talk Shows throughout the English-speaking world. Consultants to Presidents and Royalty, to the Stars of Stage, Screen and TV and to Champion Athletes, Patricia and her father Co-Authored the Bragg Health Library of Instructive, Inspiring Books that promote a healthier lifestyle, for a long, vital life.

Patricia herself is the symbol of health, perpetual youth and super energy. She is a living and sparkling example of her and her father's healthy lifestyle precepts and this she loves sharing world-wide.

A fifth-generation Californian on her mother's side, Patricia was reared by The Bragg Natural Health Method from infancy. In school, she not only excelled in athletics, but also won honors for her studies and her counseling. She is an accomplished musician and dancer . . . as well as tennis player and mountain climber . . . and the youngest woman ever to be granted a U.S. Patent. Patricia is a popular gifted Health Teacher and a dynamic, in-demand Talk Show Guest where she spreads the simple, easy-to-follow Bragg Healthy Lifestyle for everyone of all ages.

Man's body is his vehicle through life, his earthly temple . . . and the Creator wants us filled with joy & health for a long fruitful life. The Bragg Crusades of Health and Fitness (3 John 2) has carried her around the world over 13 times – spreading physical, spiritual, emotional and mental health and joy. Health is our birthright and Patricia teaches how to prevent the destruction of our health from man-made wrong habits of living.

Patricia's been a Health Consultant to American Presidents and British Royalty, to Betty Cuthbert, Australia's "Golden Girl," who holds 16 world records and four Olympic gold medals in women's track and to New Zealand's Olympic Track and Triathlete Star, Allison Roe. Among those who come to her for advice are some of Hollywood's top Stars from Clint Eastwood to the ever-youthful singing group, The Beach Boys and their families, Singing Stars of the Metropolitan Opera and top Ballet Stars. Patricia's message is of world-wide appeal to people of all ages, nationalities and walks-of-life. Those who follow The Bragg Healthy Lifestyle and attend the Bragg Crusades world-wide are living testimonials . . . like ageless, super athlete, Jack LaLanne, who at age 15 went from sickness to Total Health!

Patricia inspires you to Renew, Rejuvenate and Revitalize your life with "The Bragg Healthy Lifestyle" Books and Crusades worldwide. Millions have benefitted from these life-changing events with a longer, healthier and happier life! She loves to share with your community, organization, church groups, etc. Also, she is a perfect radio and TV talk show guest to spread the message of healthy lifestyle living. See and hear Patricia on the web: bragg.com

For Radio interview requests and info write or call (805) 968-1020
BRAGG HEALTH CRUSADES, BOX 7, SANTA BARBARA, CA 93102, USA